AF753674

AGING ISSUES, HEALTH AND FINANCIAL ALTERNATIVES SERIES

NEW DIRECTIONS IN AGING RESEARCH: HEALTH AND COGNITION

Aging Issues, Health and Financial Alternatives Series

New Directions in Aging Research: Health and Cognition
Ruby R. Brougham (Editor)
2009. ISBN: 978-1-60741-976-1

AGING ISSUES, HEALTH AND FINANCIAL ALTERNATIVES SERIES

NEW DIRECTIONS IN AGING RESEARCH: HEALTH AND COGNITION

RUBY R. BROUGHAM
EDITOR

Nova Biomedical Books
New York

Copyright © 2009 by Nova Science Publishers, Inc.

All rights reserved. No part of this book may be reproduced, stored in a retrieval system or transmitted in any form or by any means: electronic, electrostatic, magnetic, tape, mechanical photocopying, recording or otherwise without the written permission of the Publisher.

For permission to use material from this book please contact us:
Telephone 631-231-7269; Fax 631-231-8175
Web Site: http://www.novapublishers.com

NOTICE TO THE READER

The Publisher has taken reasonable care in the preparation of this book, but makes no expressed or implied warranty of any kind and assumes no responsibility for any errors or omissions. No liability is assumed for incidental or consequential damages in connection with or arising out of information contained in this book. The Publisher shall not be liable for any special, consequential, or exemplary damages resulting, in whole or in part, from the readers' use of, or reliance upon, this material.

Independent verification should be sought for any data, advice or recommendations contained in this book. In addition, no responsibility is assumed by the publisher for any injury and/or damage to persons or property arising from any methods, products, instructions, ideas or otherwise contained in this publication.

This publication is designed to provide accurate and authoritative information with regard to the subject matter covered herein. It is sold with the clear understanding that the Publisher is not engaged in rendering legal or any other professional services. If legal or any other expert assistance is required, the services of a competent person should be sought. FROM A DECLARATION OF PARTICIPANTS JOINTLY ADOPTED BY A COMMITTEE OF THE AMERICAN BAR ASSOCIATION AND A COMMITTEE OF PUBLISHERS.

Library of Congress Cataloging-in-Publication Data

New directions in aging research : health and cognition / [edited by] Ruby R. Brougham.
p. ; cm.
Includes bibliographical references and index.
ISBN 978-1-60741-976-1 (hardcover : alk. paper)
1. Senile dementia. 2. Cognition in old age. I. Brougham, Ruby R.
[DNLM: 1. Cognition Disorders. 2. Aged. 3. Aging. 4. Cognition. WT 150 N5315 2009]
RC524.N493 2009
618.97'683--dc22

2009025197

Published by Nova Science Publishers, Inc. ✝ New York

This book is dedicated to Chandra M. Mehrotra, Ph.D. who inspired, mentored, and challenged each of us to be better than we were.

Contents

Contributors

Jamila Bookwala, Ph.D., is an Associate Professor of Psychology at Lafayette College in Easton, Pennsylvania. She obtained her Ph.D. from University of Pittsburgh in the area of Social Psychology. Dr. Bookwala conducts research on the impact of family caregiving, the role of marital relationships in psychological and physical well-being during middle and late adulthood, and gender differences in health during the adulthood years. She has received grants to support her research program from the National Institute on Aging, the Midlife in the United States (MIDUS) Pilot Grant Program, the Anthony Marchionne Foundation, the Lindback Foundation, the Wisconsin Longitudinal Study Pilot Grant Program, and Lafayette College. Dr. Bookwala has published in numerous peer-reviewed journals including *Journal of Gerontology: Psychological Sciences*, *Sex Roles*, and *Journal of Aging and Health.* She serves on the editorial board of *Journals of Gerontology: Psychological Sciences*, and *The Gerontologist.*

Ruby Brougham, Ph.D., (Editor), is an Assistant Professor at Chapman University in Orange, California. She obtained her Ph.D. from the University of Southern California in the area of Adult Development and Aging. She conducts research on decision making and aging in two primary research areas. One area of research is retirement decision-making, with an emphasis on personal goals and the work environment of middle age and older adults. Another area of research concentrates on potential age differences in future time perspective and the role of future time perspective in preventive health decisions. TIAA-CREF has provided support for Dr. Brougham's work. She has published in several peer-reviewed journals including *The International Journal of Aging and Human Development, Educational Gerontology,* and *Current Psychology.*

Chih-Hung Chang, Ph.D., is an Associate Professor of Medicine and the Director of Methodology and Infometrics Section at the Buehler Center on Aging, Health and Society, Feinberg School of Medicine, Northwestern University. Dr. Chang graduated from National Chengchi University in Taiwan in 1987, where he received his bachelor's degree in Psychology. He began graduate work at the University of Chicago in 1988 and received his Ph.D. from the Committee on Research Methodology and Quantitative Psychology of the Department of Psychology in 1995. After graduation, Dr. Chang served as Assistant Professor in the Department of Psychology at Rush-Presbyterian-St. Luke's Medical Center where he held the position of Psychometrician in the Division of

Psychosocial Oncology of the Rush Cancer Institute. Prior to joining the Buehler Center, he served as Director of Psychometrics and Informatics at the Center on Outcomes, Research and Education (CORE) of Evanston Northwestern Healthcare. He was also a Research Assistant Professor in the Institute for Health Services Research and Policy Studies of Northwestern University. Dr. Chang's research interests center on the integration of methodologies and technologies to improve the quality of care and patient safety, particularly in the elderly population. He is a psychometrician with pioneering expertise in applying item response theory and computerized adaptive testing to quality of life and patient-reported outcome assessments. Dr. Chang has received grants from the National Institute of Aging (NIA), National Cancer Institute (NCI), and the National Institute of Nursing Research (NINR). He has authored numerous articles in peer-reviewed journals and serves as the editor-in-chief of the *Clinical Medicine: Geriatrics* journal and an associate editor of the *Quality of Life Research* journal

Douglas A. Hershey, Ph.D., is an Associate Professor of Psychology in the Lifespan Developmental Psychology program at Oklahoma State University. He obtained his Ph.D. in 1990 from the University of Southern California in the area of Adult Development and Aging. Dr. Hershey currently serves as Director of the Retirement Planning Research Laboratory. Dr. Hershey's work examines the development of life planning and decision- making processes in adults. He has published over three dozen articles on the topic of retirement planning, with a special interest in the cognitive, personality, and affective factors that motivate individuals to plan for the future and save for old age. For the past decade Professor Hershey has been working on the development of a comprehensive interdisciplinary model of retirement preparation. Hershey serves on the editorial board of *Certified Senior Advisor,* and he has been an *ad hoc* reviewer for numerous other journals. In 2003, Professor Hershey was appointed a Fellow of the Gerontological Society of America, and in 2007-08 he served as a Fellow-in-Residence at the Netherlands Institute for Advanced Studies in the Hague. Dr. Hershey has received support for his research from the AARP/Andrus Foundation, TIAA-CREF, the Royal Dutch Academy of Sciences, and the National Institute on Aging.

Diane Howieson, Ph.D., is a clinical neuropsychologist and Associate Professor of Neurology and Psychiatry at the Oregon Health and Science University. She obtained her board certification in 1984 from the American Board of Clinical Neuropsychology (ABPP) and serves on its Examination Committee. Her principle research focus is in the area of aging and dementia. She is an investigator in the Layton Aging and Alzheimer's Research Center at the Oregon Health and Science University. She provides evaluations of memory and other cognitive functions as well as behavior that are used for diagnosis and treatment planning for patients with known or suspected neurological diseases, particularly Alzheimer's disease and related dementias. She is an investigator with the Oregon Brain Aging Study, a longitudinal study of healthy aging in community dwelling elders age 80 years and older. She has served as Program Chair of the North American International Neuropsychological Society meeting and as Chair of the Awards Committee of the American Psychological Association Division 40 (Neuropsychology). She is a reviewer for the *Journal of the International Neuropsychological Society* and an ad-hoc reviewer for a number of other journals. She is a co-author with Dr.'s Muriel

Lezak and David Loring on *Neuropsychological Assessment*, 4th edition, Oxford University Press, 2004.

Robert Krikorian, Ph.D., is an Associate Professor in the Department of Psychiatry and Director of the Cognitive Disorders Center at the University of Cincinnati Medical Center. He earned B.A. and M.A. degrees in Philosophy from Boston University and M.A. and Ph.D. degrees in Psychology from the University of Cincinnati. He served for several years as a member of the Behavioral Medicine study section at the NIH Center for Scientific Review and is a member of the Board of Directors of the Calorie Restriction Society. He also serves as Chair of the Professional Advisory Council of the Alzheimer's Association of Cincinnati. His clinical and research interests include developmental change in cognition, the influence of health conditions on memory decline and risk for Alzheimer's disease, and interventional approaches to forestall progression of neurodegeneration. His current research involves investigations of the effects of novel, non-pharmaceutical interventions on neurocognitive function in older adults with early memory decline and the effects of such interventions on inflammatory and metabolic mediators of cognitive function. Funding for his research has come from the National Institute on Aging, the National Center for Complementary and Alternative Medicine, and from a number of foundation and industry sources.

Maureen Schmitter-Edgecombe, Ph.D., is a Professor in the Department of Psychology at Washington State University. She received her Ph.D. in Clinical Psychology with specialized training in Neuropsychology from The University of Memphis in 1994. She has built a strong research program in clinical neuropsychology, rehabilitation, and traumatic brain injury. She is currently conducting studies with early-stage dementia patients and the evaluation of memory compensation techniques and use of "smart" environment technologies. This research is directed towards extending the everyday independence of people with dementia, decreasing caregiver burden, and increasing quality of life for both members of the care dyad. She has received significant grants from the National Institute of Neurological and Stroke Disorders, the National Institute of Child Health and Human Development, and the Life Sciences Discovery Fund. Her research has been widely published in national and international peer-reviewed journals.

Mitzi M. Schumacher, Ph.D., is a full Professor in the Behavioral Science Department of the College of Medicine at the University of Kentucky. Dr. Schumacher received her degree in social psychology from the Ohio State University in 1986. Before becoming a faculty member at the University of Kentucky she completed two post doctoral fellowship; the first a National Institute of Mental Health fellowship in medical behavioral science, the second a National Institute on Aging fellowship in gerontology. Her primary research interests in aging and cognition concentrate on potential age differences in decision-making processes that lead to the use of heuristics. While her early research examined basic cognitive processes, her most recent research examines the collaborative cognition underlying shared decision-making and the contextual influences inherent to making medical decisions. She also has research interests in medical education and gender issues in academe. Dr. Schumacher has received grants from the National Institutes of Health and National Institute on Aging. She has published in numerous peer-reviewed journals including *Journal of Cancer Education*, *Journal of Gerontology: Psychological Sciences*, and *Psychology and Aging.*

Lisa Sparks, Ph.D., is the Director of Graduate Studies in Health Communication, Presidential Research Fellow in Health and Risk, and full Professor of Communication at Chapman University in Orange, California. She obtained her Ph.D. from the University of Oklahoma in the area of Communication with cognate areas in Health Risk Communication and Aging and Life Span Development. Before becoming a faculty member at Chapman University, Dr. Sparks served as an Associate Professor and Director of Graduate Studies of the Department of Communication at George Mason University in Fairfax, Virginia. She also served as a Cancer Research Fellow at the National Cancer Research Institute (NCI) and National Institute of Health (NIH) in Bethesda, Maryland. Currently, she serves as a Full Member of the Chao Family Comprehensive Cancer Research Center (NCI-Designated) at the University of California, Irvine. Dr. Sparks's research interests include the areas of health and risk/crisis communication, health literacy, patient-centered communication, and aging and lifespan development. She has received support for research from the National Institute of Health (NIH), Glaxo-Wellcome, Inc., and the Robert Wood Johnson Foundation. Since 1995, Dr. Sparks has published more than 40 student-centered handbooks, instructor's resource manuals, and teaching ideas for general education basic courses. She has published in numerous peer-reviewed journals including *Health Communication*, *Patient Education Counseling*, and the *Journal of Applied Communication Research.*

Introduction

Ruby R. Brougham
Chapman University, Orange, California, USA

First and foremost, the National Institute on Aging made this book possible. Many of the contributors to this book attended the Institute on Research in Psychology of Aging in the summer of 2003. The Institute brought together psychologists with a wide variety of expertise: to learn about advanced methods in research methodology, to identify research problems and to identify solutions for an aging population. A community of scholars dedicated to advancing teaching and research in the area of aging was formed at the Institute. This book is a community effort and reflects our current research and future directions for research with an emphasis on addressing and solving the timely problems of aging, health, and cognition.

The first chapter in the book investigates the role of lifestyle habits, particularly nutrition, physical activity, and stress in neurocognitive decline and dementia. Krikorian provides compelling evidence for a link between brain health and the specific chronic disease states of hypertension, hyperinsulinemia, and cortisol abnormalities. This decline in brain health is not universal. For example, certain populations, such as the Japanese living in Okinawa, have few chronic diseases, few cognitive or physical declines, and extraordinary longevity. The Okinawans are dissimilar to developed societies with respect to stress, socialization characteristics, demand for physical activity, and diet. Thus, Krikorian argues for a lifestyle intervention that prevents and reduces cognitive decline. In particular, an environmental intervention that includes a reduction or elimination of refined sugar and carbohydrates in diets, increased physical activity, and greater focus on stress reduction (e.g., through social support). Furthermore, it is noted that effective pharmaceutical treatment for dementia is not currently available (pharmaceutical treatments provide time-limited, symptomatic improvement for about 50% of patients) and existing pharmaceutical treatments for chronic disease may not reduce the risk for deterioration of brain functioning. Krikorian concludes that aging is strongly linked to disease, and a greater understanding of the nature of the relationship between aging and disease is crucial in the context of guiding research intended to alter health outcomes in late life.

The second chapter of the book focuses on the relationship between Body Mass Index (BMI) and psychological well-being. In particular, Bookwala and colleague examine whether gender has an influence on the relationship between Body Mass Index and psychological well-being. Using a sample of 3,322 middle-age adults they found that overweight and obese women reported decreased well-being (lower positive relations with others, lower environmental mastery, and lower personal growth) than normal weight women. However, men's psychological well-being did not differ by body weight. Furthermore, normal weight women report better psychological well-being than normal weight men. Bookwala and colleague propose that poorer psychological well-being may place overweight individuals at an elevated risk for a mood or anxiety disorder. They conclude that stigma and gender differentiated culture norms may explain the gender differences in psychological well-being for overweight adults. Bookwala and colleague recommend that future research continue to explore the relationship between psychological well-being and body weight.

Chapters three and four propose innovative cognitive rehabilitation interventions for older adults with early stage Alzheimer's disease and Mild Cognitive Impairment. Schmitter-Edgecombe and colleagues present pioneering work on a combined cognitive rehabilitation and dyadic (aimed at working with both patient and caregiver) notebook intervention for early stage Alzheimer's patients. The 7-week memory notebook intervention incorporated both behavioral learning principals and educational strategies. The intervention consisted of modeling, psychoeducation (e.g. increase understanding of how changes in the brain affect behavior), and the completion of activities directed by therapists. Benefits of the notebook intervention included patients reporting greater confidence in their support systems, caregivers reporting less depression, and improvements in memory compensation. Schmitter-Edgecombe and colleagues suggests that one important direction for future research is the continued empirical validation of blended dyadic cognitive rehabilitation interventions (that include patient and caregiver) for Alzheimer's disease.

In chapter four, Seelye, Howieson and colleagues report on two behavioral interventions designed to improve daily functioning, mood, and quality of life for individuals with Mild Cognitive Impairment (MCI). The intervention also combined cognitive rehabilitation with dyadic intervention (patient and study partner). One intervention used an electronic memory device to compensate for memory impairment; while the other intervention used cognitive-behavioral therapy techniques to manage emotional reactions and used non-electronic memory aids with errorless learning instruction to compensate for memory impairment. No prior studies have tested the feasibility of using electronic device interventions with MCI patients. The results showed: 1) that the electronic memory device intervention resulted in improvements in patients' functioning in daily activities, and 2) the cognitive behavioral therapy intervention resulted in patients' reports of better memory and greater use of memory compensation strategies. Although patients report that the intervention was a positive experience and they benefited from the experience, they did not report an improvement in quality of life or mood after the intervention. Since most patients reported a high quality of life and mood at the onset of training, it is recommended that future testing of the interventions use a group with greater reported variability in mood and quality of life. In support of the dyadic component of this intervention, study partners were found to be important sources for role modeling, helpful in assisting patients' with learning of new skills, and empathetic in responding to patients' emotional reactions to memory failure. Recommendations for development, validation, and accessibility of behavioral interventions for patients' with MCI are suggested as directions for future research.

In the fifth chapter of the book, Chang presents an innovative methodology combined with advanced technology to assess pain in geriatric cancer patients. Pain in geriatric cancer patients is a pressing issue given the demographic trends pointing to an increasing population of older cancer patients, for whom pain will be a significant consequence. Since the experience of pain is subjective and multidimensional (including physical, psychological, social, cultural, and spiritual components) it is difficult to assess and effectively measure pain. Although several high quality instruments exist to measure pain, none are comprehensive. As a remedy to pain assessment difficulties, Chang proposes an innovative technology: Pain Computerized Adaptive Testing. Pain Computerized Adaptive Testing is a multipurpose assessment program with the capability to store pain items, administer fixed-length and adaptive tests, and generate reports in diverse settings (such as homes and assisted living) using advanced technologies (e.g. Personal Digital Phones, iPhone) and Item Response Theory Methodology. Furthermore, future directions for pain research include using the Pain Computerized Adaptive Testing for other populations and validating the usability of this technology.

In chapter six, Sparks and colleague review the relationship between health literacy, cognition, and emotion in older adults. Health literacy includes the concepts of accessing and understanding health information and services, with a comprehensive skill set of literacy that potentially includes visual (graphs and charts), computer (operate and search), information (obtain and apply relevant information), and numeracy (calculate and reason numerically) skills required to make appropriate health decisions. Current reports from the American Medical Association suggest that older adults, those over the age of 65, are the most vulnerable to the health consequences caused by poor health literacy. Older adults who have low health literacy are likely to have difficulty describing symptoms, providing an accurate health history, and understanding the health diagnosis and treatment recommended by their health care provider. The current chapter identifies and discusses the cognitive and emotional changes that impact information processing, communication, and decision-making; and place older adults at greater risk for problems in clinical (e.g., diagnosis, treatment, and medication), prevention (maintaining and improving health), and navigation (e.g., understanding the rights and responsibilities associated with health care) of the health care system. The current chapter also identifies and discusses the diversity of the baby boom generation (those born between 1946 and 1964), the use of the Internet to tailor health care recommendations, and the adaptation of health care providers to their changing roles as critical directions for future research. A specific research agenda is presented at the end of the chapter.

Chapters seven and eight explore the relationship between decision-making and aging. In chapter seven, Schumacher and colleague examine the relationship between age and decision-making under conditions of time constraints. In the aging literature, it is well established that a number of basic cognitive abilities, including information processing speed, decline with age. However, less is known about how these declines impact the decision-making of older adults. A greater understanding of the adaptations made by older adults' under conditions of time constraints would inform the development of decision aids that could assist older adults with complex decisions that have to be made under time pressure. Schumacher and colleague report on two studies that examine how older adults use adaptive strategies to make real-world decisions under time constraints. In study 1, under conditions of time constraint for decision-making, old and young adults used different decision strategies to make similar decisions. Young adults were found to speed up their decision processing and decrease their information use, while older adults decreased their information use and increased the organization of their information searches. In study 2, under conditions of fixed time for reviewing decision information, young and older adults were found to make different decisions. In terms of decision strategies for study 2, young adults lowered their decision criteria, while older adults increased the organization of their information searches. The results of both studies are discussed in terms of older adults' adaptation to limitations in information processing when making complex real-world decisions. Suggestions for future directions in research include a greater understanding of the relationship between stress and older adults' decision-making.

In chapter 8, Brougham and colleague review the relationship between future time perspective, income, health and age. Promoting preventive health behaviors and retirement savings is critical to the well-being of all Americans given the demographic trend in the United States towards a large number of older adults using social services (e.g., Social Security and Medicare) and fewer working adults to pay for those services. Brougham and colleague propose that a better understanding of future time perspective, that is, how future experiences and consequences are evaluated and compared to the present, is one critical factor for understanding decision-making. Many decisions involve consequences (benefits and costs) that unfold over time. Preventive health decisions (e.g., exercise, nutrition, tobacco use) and financial decisions involve a trade-offs between benefits (e.g., eat several cookies now) and costs (e.g., gain weight). Future time perspective encompasses cognitive processes (e.g., planning, regulation of behavior), emotion (e.g., anxiety) and motivation (e.g., values and goals). The chapter reviews the fundamental concepts of intertemporal choice, time discounting and related empirical research. New and emerging areas of research in future time perspective including future representation of events, age and life events, and emotion are discussed. Specific determinants (e.g., anxiety) that tip decisions toward greater concern for future versus present consequences are identified. Furthermore applications of research for interventions are proposed.

In the final chapter, Hershey and colleague examine the content, structure, and process aspects of individuals' retirement goals. Although goal-setting has been identified as a fundamental motivation for behavior, few empirical investigations of retirement goals have been published. Retirement is a stage of life often marked by novel developmental tasks, opportunities, and freedom. It is a time when the "young old" can pursue new directions or focus on long-standing interests, which previously may not have been possible due to career commitments and family responsibilities. Retirement is recognized as the last stage of occupational development but the corresponding goals of this stage have not been well identified. The current study included 184 working adults who ranged in age from 20 - 64 years of age. With regard to the content of retirement goals, individuals rated the importance of being happy, financial independence, good health, and time spent with family members as important. A two-factor model of self-oriented goals and goals involving others was identified as a plausible structure for retirement goals. As for the process aspects of individual's retirement goals, goal striving (the amount of thought and effort allocated to achieving a goal) was found to predict goal expectancy (the likelihood that the goal would be achieved). Age differences in retirement goals were not found. Hershey and colleague suggest that this may be the result of a culture that indoctrinates individuals to begin thinking about retirement at an early age. Suggested directions for future research include examining the diversity of goals among people of different races and ethnicities and longitudinal studies that reveal pertinent information about how retirement goals change with age.

In: New Directions in Aging Research
Editor: Ruby R. Brougham, pp. 1-23
ISBN 978-1-60741-976-1
© 2009 Nova Science Publishers, Inc.

Chapter 1

Health Factors and Cognitive Aging

Robert Krikorian*
Department of Psychiatry, University of Cincinnati, Cincinnati, Ohio, USA

Abstract

General health is linked to brain health, and age-related diseases are associated with neurocognitive decline and dementia. Alzheimer's disease (AD) might be conceptualized as one of the diseases of civilization in the same sense as hypertension and type 2 diabetes. Diseases of aging are highly prevalent in developed and developing cultures and, to a large extent, reflect the substantial departure of contemporary lifestyle from that of pre-agricultural epochs during which human physiological adaptations evolved. Endocrine dysregulation, cardiovascular risks, and metabolic abnormalities, the most prevalent age-related health conditions observed in western societies, have interactive effects in contributing to general health disorders as well as to neurodegeneration. Compensatory hyperinsulinemia, in particular, produces a myriad of direct and indirect effects on neurocognitive function. Effective treatment for dementia is not available, and existing pharmaceutical therapies for diseases of aging may not significantly lower risk. Accordingly, prevention represents the optimal approach to this growing public health problem. It has been proposed that the identification of individuals in the earliest phases of neurodegeneration may provide an opportunity for intervention to forestall progression. Risks for dementia, in particular metabolic abnormalities, are amenable to behaviorally-mediated interventions involving alteration of lifestyle factors. Such preventive approaches offer the possibility of substantially reducing the prevalence of dementing conditions such as Alzheimer's disease while improving general health.

* Correspondence: Robert Krikorian, PhD, Department of Psychiatry, University of Cincinnati Academic Health Center, PO Box 670559, Cincinnati, OH 45267-0559; robert.krikorian@uc.edu

Introduction

This chapter will focus on the relationship of age-related health disorders to acquired cognitive decline and dementia, principally Alzheimer's disease. Caloric abundance, sanitation, and medical intervention have served to increase average lifespan in developed countries. However, for many older adults, health span has not increased with lifespan and late life involves living with disease. Approximately 80% of individuals over the age of 65 have one or more chronic medical conditions (La Rue, 1992), and, ironically, it may be that many of the environmental factors in developed countries that contribute to increasing average life span also contribute to late life disease. In western societies older adults survive for many years with chronic health conditions that diminish functional capability and quality of life. Important examples, among several, include hypertension and insulin resistance. The incidence of high blood pressure increases linearly with age beginning in middle life and is ubiquitous in the elderly. The prevalence of hypertension in the United States for individuals aged 65 and older is 70% (Centers for Disease Control and Prevention, 2004). In addition, it is estimated that 50% of individuals 60 years and older have insulin resistance (Craft, 2005), the precursor to type 2 diabetes, which itself has increased in prevalence in recent years to 23.8% of the population over 60 (Centers for Disease Control and Prevention, 2004).

Table 1 contains a list of several chronic diseases of aging. These are the conditions that contribute to functional decline and suffering with aging and ultimately to death. Note that Alzheimer's disease is included on this list. It is our contention that, to a large extent, these diseases not only represent decline in general health but also are associated with cognitive disorders and neurodegeneration. Virtually all of these conditions develop over a time frame of several years and are the result of long-standing maladaptation of fundamental physiological processes that influence general health and brain health.

Table 1. Diseases of Civilization

Insulin resistance
Hypertension
Type 2 diabetes
Heart disease
Osteoporosis
Sarcopenia
Arthritis
Cancer
Memory disorders (Alzheimer's disease)

Categories of Cognitive Aging

While wisdom and acquired knowledge can enhance function with aging, co-occurring decline of information processing abilities, in particular working memory and long-term memory impairments, contributes to functional deterioration and, ultimately, to disability. We might classify older adults with respect to cognitive status in four broad categories.

Successful aging is characterized by comparatively little functional decline mentally or physically and extraordinary longevity, often into the 10th decade and beyond (Rowe and Kahn, 1998). In most cultures genuine successful aging occurs in an exceedingly small minority of exceptional elderly adults. Recent cohorts of older adults in Okinawa, Japan may represent the best example of such populations. Proportionally, the Okinawan culture has more centenarians than any developed country including other areas of Japan. The preservation of function among the oldest old in this cohort appears to be consequences of both particular lifestyle habits (Willcox, Willcox, Todoriki, Curb, and Suzuki, 2006) and favorable genetic factors (Willcox, Willcox, He, Curb and Suzuki, 2006). Prevalence of dementia among older Okinawans is reduced relative to mainland Japan and the United States (Kokmen, Bear, O'Brien and Kruland, 1996; Ogura, et al., 1995), marking the direct association of general health and brain health. These observations suggest a highly positive gene-environment interaction for elderly Okinawans. The Okinawan environment has been dissimilar in comparison with developed societies with respect to stress and socialization characteristics, demand for physical activity, and diet (Willcox, et al., 2006). In contrast, exceedingly high rates of disease are present in the very old in other western societies (Anderson-Ranberg, Schroll, and Jeune, 2001), and a review of several survey studies of North American communities observed rates of dementia in centenarians ranging from 75% to 85% (Perls, 2004). Such data would indicate that the Okinawan cohort is, indeed, comparatively highly successful with respect to longevity as well as preservation of general health and mental function, perhaps resulting from genetic factors favoring longevity in the context of an optimal environment.

The Kitavan people represent another interesting and instructive example of longevity and absence of chronic, age-related illness. Kitava is one of the Trobriand Islands in Papua New Guinea, and Kitava represents one of the few remaining cultures with dietary habits and general lifestyle approximating that of pre-agricultural people. Medical surveys of the Kitavan population indicate dramatic health divergence from western societies such as absence of cardiovascular disease and risk factors and absence of metabolic disorders. Further, there is no dementia or memory impairment in late life and older adults experience good quality of life and sustain physical activity until very near death (Lindeberg, Eliasson, Lindahl, and Ahren, 1999; Lindeberg and Lundh, 1993). It is noteworthy that level of physical activity is only slightly greater than that of westerners and that 80% of the adult population are smokers. However, the major difference appears to be diet, which consists chiefly of tubers, fruits, vegetables, fish, and coconuts.

Age-Associated Memory Impairment (AAMI) refers to so-called normal age-related cognitive decline or benign senescent forgetfulness (Crook. et al., 1986; Neilsen, Lolk, and Kragk-Sorenson, 1998). It involves gradual occurrence of forgetfulness in the context of relatively little functional difficulty. Older adults with AAMI tend to have subjective memory complaints and to perform more poorly than younger cohorts on objective memory tests (Crook, et al., 1986). However, there are indications that even purportedly benign decline observed in AAMI can reflect significant neurodegeneration for a subset of individuals. Older adults with subjective memory complaints show degradation in medial temporal lobe that is similar, although not as extensive as that observed in subjects with Mild Cognitive Impairment and Alzheimer's disease (Goldman and Morris, 2001). The medial temporal lobe contains several structures including the hippocampus and parahippocampal cortices that are essential for episodic learning and memory (Squire, Stark and Clark, 2004). Also, longitudinal investigation has shown a tripling of risk for progression to dementia for those categorized as having AAMI (Saykin, et al., 2006).

Mild Cognitive Impairment (MCI; Petersen 2003) is a recently coined term that refers to age-related memory decline that often is the first clinical manifestation of dementia, in particular, Alzheimer's disease (AD). MCI, and similar constructs such as Cognitive Impairment, no Dementia (Ebly, Hogan, and Parkad, 1995) identify individuals with substantially elevated risk of dementia (Chertkow, et al., 2008). Clinic-based, longitudinal studies have documented rates of progression from MCI to AD ranging from 10% to 15% annually (Bowen, et al. 1997; Flicker, Ferris, and Reisberg, 1991), with progression over a six-year period as great as 80% (Petersen, et al., 1999; 2001). Although one would expect lower risk in community as opposed to clinic samples, the incremental increase in magnitude of risk associated with MCI clearly is large.

Dementia occurs in about 14% of the elderly population in the United States (Plassman, et al., 2007). Alzheimer's disease (AD) is the most prevalent form of dementia, accounting for between 60% and 80% of dementia cases (Alzheimer's Association, 2008). Late onset or sporadic AD is much more common than the early onset form, which occurs before age 65. AD involves progressive neurodegeneration with prominent memory disorder in the earlier phases. Classic cortical function deficits involving language, visual-spatial function, and praxis (ability to perform skilled movements) become prominent in the later stages when there is global impairment of functional capability. The absence of disease modifying treatment options along with population statistics projections indicate that there will be an extraordinary increase in the number of individuals with AD over the next several decades.

Alzheimer's disease involves degeneration of specific brain regions including hippocampal and parahippocampal structures in the medial temporal lobe and areas of neocortex. Figure 1 is a schematic representation depicting information transfer between the neocortical association areas and medical temporal lobe. Association cortexes for each of the major sensory processing systems have projections to areas that are transitional between the neocortex and hippocampus. These centers send outputs to the entorhinal cortex, which transmits the information to the hippocampal formation where memory consolidation is mediated. Layer 2 of the entorhinal cortex is called the preforant path, one of the most vulnerable structures in the brain.

Neurogenesis, the process of creating new neurons, which continues throughout life, occurs in the hippocampus (Gage, Kempermann, Palmer, Peterson, and Ray, 1998) and, to a lesser extent, in neocortex (Gould, Reeves, Graziano, and Gross, 1999). Brain regions involved in AD are important for problem-solving, behavioral adaptation, and new learning, and they may be the most plastic with respect to both function and structure. On the other hand, these brain regions are quite vulnerable to the interactive effects of aging and disease conditions. The entorhinal cortex is the site of the earliest degeneration in Alzheimer's disease (de Leon, et al., 2001).

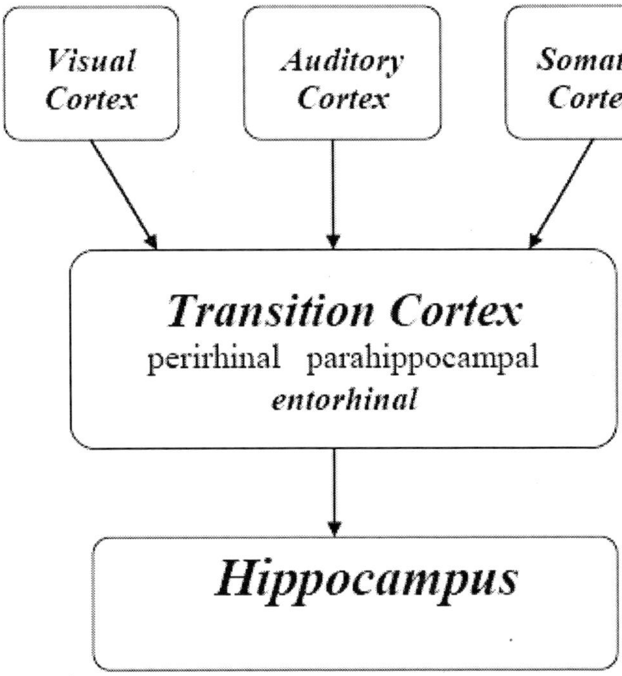

Figure 1. Information transfer between neocortical association areas and hippocampus.

General Health and Brain Health

As we have suggested, general health is linked to brain health. It is noteworthy that cognitive function is related to systemic disease at any age. As examples, young diabetics have poorer memory function than non-diabetic children (Hershey, et al., 2005), and higher consumption of refined carbohydrates is associated with lower IQ in children (Lester, Thatcher, and Monroe-Lord, 1982). Also, elevated blood pressure in middle age predicts poorer cognition in old age (Swan, Carmelli, and La Rue, 1998). With aging, the influence of health factors on cognitive function is magnified. The diseases identified in Table 1 are among the most prevalent health conditions observed in developed societies. These disease conditions might be conceptualized as a cluster of disorders generated by common aberrant processes rather than as disparate conditions with distinct or exclusive pathophysiological mechanisms. It is useful to examine how health factors discretely influence cognitive-cerebral function but with a view toward appreciating the shared mechanisms underlying these factors, despite the fact that they often are purported to be independent.

Stress and Cortisol Exposure

The concept stress implies a demand for organism adaptation. In broad terms, stressful experiences can be distinguished with respect to intensity and duration, factors that have implications for whether their effects are adverse or beneficial. Allostatic response systems are by design adapted to manage short-term moderate stress. Time-limited, moderate intensity stressors tend not to damage physiological systems. Indeed, brief stress exposure tends to produce beneficial physiological responses, as is the case with bouts of moderate exercise and short-term calorie deprivation. On the other hand, chronic stress exposure can lead to elevated basal levels of hormones that contribute to health disorders such as hypertension and obesity.

Stress hormones play a role in a variety of aging processes including cognitive aging (McEwen, de Leon, Lupien, and Meaney, 1999). Cortisol is a primary human stress response hormone and is of particular interest because of dose-dependent effects on memory function and its potential effects on the integrity of the hippocampal and neocortical brain structures that are vulnerable in dementia (Lupien, et al., 2005). Cortisol is an adrenal hormone regulated by the hypothalamic-pituitary-adrenal (HPA) axis as well as by feedback inhibition mediated by receptors located in the temporal lobe and neocortex. It is of interest to note that the distribution of cortisol receptors in these brain regions parallels that of insulin receptors. Cortisol is released to help re-establish homeostasis in response to adaptational demands. Cortisol has several effects, among them releasing energy from storage sites through several mechanisms that serve to elevate plasma glucose, increasing blood pressure, and dampening immune system response. Insulin and cortisol have opposing effects in that the energy releasing actions of cortisol counteracts the energy storage action of insulin. In addition, cortisone, a cortisol metabolite, strongly inhibits insulin secretion. Cortisol, in conjunction with other stress hormones, epinephrine and norepinephrine, also facilitates emotional memory formation through actions in the hippocampus and amygdala. Such effects represent normal physiological processes in the context of time-limited stress exposure. However, these same actions account for negative effects of long-term stress and prolonged, excess cortisol secretion. An important issue in this regard is that receptor over-exposure to cortisol induces receptor resistance (as is the case with excess insulin receptor exposure, as described below) and can lead to increasingly greater cortisol secretion and, ultimately, to cognitive dysfunction and hippocampal atrophy.

Impaired regulation of cortisol secretion has been shown to be a factor that increases vulnerability to age-related cerebral deterioration. Increased susceptibility to neuronal apoptosis and decreased glucose transport are among the cellular and molecular mechanisms of action associated with chronic exposure to high levels of cortisol (Porter and Landfield, 1998). Also, long-term exposure to elevated cortisol in conjunction with actions of excitatory amino acid neurotransmitters (glutamate) contribute to a reduction of glucocorticoid receptors and consequent loss of inhibitory feedback regulation of cortisol secretion leading to progressive damage to hippocampus and neocortex (Brown, Tush, and McEwen, 1999). Susceptibility to these processes has been shown to be greater for the elderly and for those with longer periods of elevated cortisol exposure (Lupien, et al., 1999).

HPA axis dysfunction and chronic stress, both reflected in elevated basal cortisol levels, have been implicated in Alzheimer's disease (Davis, et al., 1986; Wilson, et al., 2005), especially in the early stages (Sanwick, et al., 1998). A majority of elderly individuals in whom there is an association between elevated cortisol and hippocampal atrophy are diagnosed subsequently with Alzheimer's disease (Deleon, et al., 1993). Such evidence suggests a relationship between early cognitive decline and AD mediated in part by glucocorticoid actions. Elderly adults with chronic elevations of cortisol show reductions in hippocampal volume and deficits on spatial memory and problem solving tasks, again, suggesting cortisol-related hippocampal deterioration and cognitive dysfunction (Lupien, et al., 1998). Longitudinal studies have demonstrated that older adults with chronically higher basal cortisol levels show relatively deficient memory performance and decreased hippocampal volume, early signs of incipient Alzheimer's disease (Lupien, et al., 2005). Furthermore, preliminary data indicate that cortisol infusion dampens the beneficial effects of exogenous insulin administration on memory function in patients with Alzheimer's disease (Reger, et al., 2004). In animal models, glucocorticoids increase beta-amyloid and tau pathology (Green, Billings, Roozendaal, McGaugh, and LaFerla, 2006), suggesting another mechanism by which cortisol over-exposure may contribute to neurodegeneration. Young patients with Cushing's syndrome are exposed to high levels of cortisol for periods of months to years and exhibit decreased hippocampal volume. Treatment of Cushing's syndrome resulting in lowered cortisol levels is associated with increased hippocampal volume and improved memory ability in direct proportion to the extent of cortisol lowering (Starkman, et al., 2000; Starkman, Giordani, Gebarski, and Schteingart, 2003). Accordingly, reductions of cortisol, even after long periods of excess exposure, can produce beneficial adaptations in brain and improvement in cognitive function, marking the cerebral sensitivity to this hormone. Interestingly, maintenance of physiological levels of cortisol also appears to be necessary for memory function. Pharmaceutical suppression of cortisol in older adults with normal basal cortisol levels impairs memory function, and this effect is reversible with cortisol replacement (Lupien, et al., 2002). These effects were not obtained in subjects with long-standing elevations of basal cortisol, implying that the hippocampal damage associated with excessive cortisol exposure may not respond to this manipulation in vulnerable older adults.

Social relationships are important with respect to stress mediation. Of course, consistent exposure to difficult interpersonal relationships will induce chronic stress (Seeman and McEwen, 1996). However, gratifying and supportive relationships represent some of the most fundamental ways of ameliorating stress. Even simple interpersonal interaction as well as social support serves to increase psychological resiliency and reduce cortisol levels in response to stress in animal models (Coppola, Granin, and Enns, 2006) and in humans (Ditzen, et al., 2008; Heinrichs, Baumgarten, Kirschbaum, and Ehlert, 2003). In addition, it has been established that over extended intervals there is an inverse relationship between level of social support and basal cortisol, even with level of stress controlled (Rosal, King, Ma, and Reed, 2004). Thirty percent of older adults have elevated cortisol levels, and the single factor that seems to differentiate those with increased cortisol from those without is the absence of social support (Lupien, et al., 2005). Animal and human data indicate that the social environment, in particular the quality of social relationships with respect to support and gratification characteristics, influence glucocorticoid expression. While supportive social involvement decreases cortisol release in humans, nonsupportive interactions and the absence of support increase HPA reactivity and cortisol secretion (Seeman and McEwen, 1996).

Social engagement appears to be directly related to risk for dementia. In a prospective Swedish study, more than 1200 elderly, non-demented individuals were evaluated initially and again three years later with respect to cognitive status (Fratiglioni, Wang, Ericsson,

Maytan, and Winblad, 2000). In addition, level of socialization at baseline was assessed in terms of marital status, contact with children, and contact with friends and other relatives. Extent of socialization was indexed as the number of social contacts. Extent of social involvement predicted progression to dementia, as the rate of AD at three-year follow up varied directly with socialization. For those with the lowest level of social involvement (living alone, no children, and no close friend/relative), the incidence of AD was 16%. For those with limited involvement, the incidence was 7%, while moderately and extensively involved individuals had dementia rates of 5% and 2%, respectively. These effects were independent of age, gender, educational level, depression, and cognitive status at baseline. Thus, social involvement seems to be an important predictor of AD, independent of other known demographic risks, most likely mediated through the stress response system.

Cardiovascular Risks

Hypertension (HTN) is associated with cognitive decline in the context of cerebrovascular disease but also appears to be an independent risk for Alzheimer's disease in the absence of other health conditions (Skoog, et al., 2003). In the United States, the estimated prevalence of elevated blood pressure increases linearly with age beginning in midlife. For all adults aged 65 and older, the prevalence of hypertension is 70% (Centers for Disease Control and Prevention, 2004). Several studies have documented an association of hypertension with cognitive deficit in untreated and recently diagnosed adults, in those removed from antihypertensive treatment (Alves de Moraes, Szklo, Knopman, and Sato, 2002; Elias, Elias, Sullivan, Wolf, and D'Agostino, 2003; Madden and Blumenthal, 1998; Raz, Rodrigue, and Acher, 2003), and in older adults with treatment resistant HTN (Brady, Spiro, and Gaziano, 2005; Swan, Carmelli, and Larue, 1998). While there are some indications of benefit from antihypertensive medications (Dufouil, et al., 2005), studies examining the effects of treatment have been mixed (Applegate, et al., 1994; Murray, et al., 2002), and intervention with medication may not confer protection against cerebral pathology (Muldoon, et al., 2002). On balance, it is not clear whether antihypertensive treatment is protective with respect to long-term cognitive decline, produces cognitive impairment in its own right, or has no effect. It is plausible that antihypertensive treatment does not protect against cerebral pathology because these drugs reduce blood pressure by targeting downstream mechanisms that do not affect the more fundamental processes that cause both blood pressure elevation and cerebral degeneration. Merely lowering blood pressure in this manner may not affect the pathophysiology of cognitive decline associated with hypertension. There is empirical support for the notion that HTN is caused by hyperinsulinemia (Goff, Zaccaro, Hofner, and Saad, 2003).

Vascular risk factors are most often discussed with respect to their effects on cardiovascular disease, cerebrovascular disease, and stroke. However, these also are prominent factors in Alzheimer's disease. Neuropathology studies indicate that 60% to 90% of cases of AD show cerebrovascular pathology (Kalaria, 2000) and ischemia-related white matter changes, which are strongly linked to hypertension, are observed in nearly all cases of AD, even those screened to exclude patients with clinically apparent cerebrovascular disease

(Hofman, et al., 1997; Nagy et al., 1998). Also, about 33% of cases diagnosed with cerebrovascular dementia show Alzheimer's type pathological changes (Ballard, et al., 2000; Pasquier, Leya, and Scheltens, 1998). Not surprisingly, then, vascular risk factors such as hypertension and elevated homocysteine level are risks for AD (Breteler, 2000; Kalaria, 2000), and there are indications that cardiovascular disease is an etiological factor in the development of AD pathology (Farkas, De Vos, Steur, and Luiten, 2000). For example, cholesterol metabolism and apolipoprotein E (APOE) in the brain are regulated by amyloid precursor protein (Lui, et al., 2007), and the epsilon (ε) 4 allele of the APOE gene is now established as a risk for Alzheimer's disease (Holtzman, et al., 2000; Zerbinatti and Bu, 2006)

As noted, hypertension is highly prevalent in the older adult population and appears to be a significant independent risk for cognitive decline and dementia. Figure 2 shows memory performance of a group of 93 post-menopausal women systematically assessed for subjective memory complaints.

None was demented and all were functioning independently, albeit with reduced efficiency because of mild memory difficulty. Those with stroke and other neurological condition and major psychiatric disease were excluded. Memory was assessed with a paired associate learning task that is sensitive to age-related memory change and predictive of risk for further decline and dementia (Krikorian, 1996; 2006). Controlling for age, those with hypertension performed more poorly on the memory task, even in this relatively homogeneous sample of older women with common age-associated memory impairment. Such episodic memory impairment is characteristic of early neurodegeneration (Backman, Jones, Berger, Laukka, and Small, 2005; Petersen, et al., 1994), and performance on this type of memory task can anticipate future decline in those without clinically evident dementia (Spaan, Raaijmakers, and Jonder, 2005). Accordingly, those with hypertension appear to have greater risk for eventual progression to dementia.

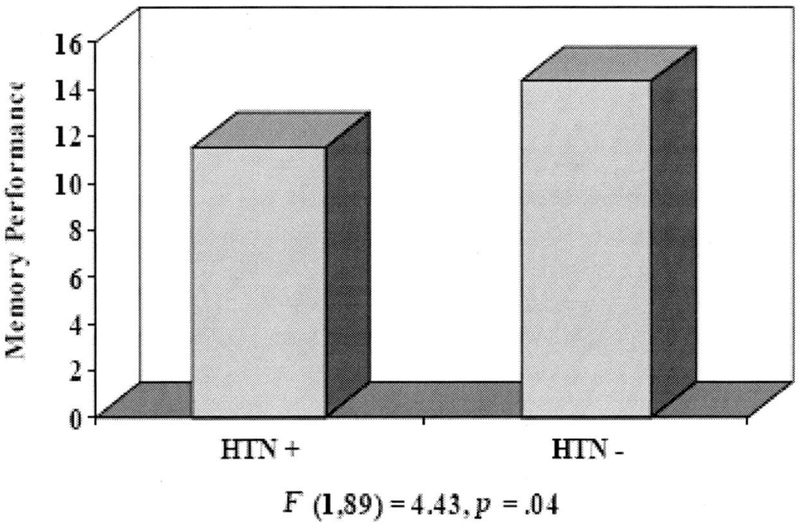

Figure 2. Hypertensive women with subjective memory complaints demonstrated poorer memory performance than those without hypertension. HTN+ = presence of hypertension. HTN- = absence of hypertension.

Metabolic Disorders

Hyperinsulinemia and the related cluster of disorders of insulin resistance syndrome are common in older adults. Hyperinsulinemia, in particular is often unrecognized, even in the context of obesity, hypertension, and elevated triglycerides. Gut peptides released in response to glucose elevations in plasma stimulate secretion of insulin from the pancreas. Chronic consumption of high glycemic, low fiber foods can lead to insulin receptor resistance and decreased receptor signaling. Because of resistance and receptor inefficiency, glucose lowering by insulin is less effective, and the pancreas secretes additional insulin to overcome tissue resistance. This compensatory hyperinsulinemia, which *de facto* results from long-standing elevated insulin levels, maintains normal glucose but is the basis for characteristic metabolic disturbances that have been recognized as part of the metabolic syndrome or insulin resistance syndrome (Reaven, 1988; 1994). In addition to hyperinsulinemia, the syndrome entails hypertension, increased waist circumference, and elevated triglycerides (Shaw, Hall, and Williams, 2005). The occurrence of compensatory hyperinsulinemia and metabolic syndrome increase with age. Diagnostic criteria for metabolic syndrome vary and population statistics differ to some extent. Estimates of the prevalence in the United States range from 20% (Scuteri, et al., 2004) to 35% (Resnick, et al., 2003), but because surveys tend to include young and middle aged adults, the prevalence in older adults certainly is much greater (Shaw, Hall, and Williams, 2005). It is estimated that about 50% of adults over age 60 are insulin resistant (Craft, 2005). Hyperinsulinemia is the precursor to type 2 diabetes, which occurs when the pancreas fails to maintain insulin at higher levels sufficient to overcome tissue resistance.

Compensatory hyperinsulinemia is directly related to dietary habits. Glycemic load is the primary factor. Figure 3 shows the carbohydrate and fiber concentrations of different categories of carbohydrate foods and food products available in western societies. Pre-agricultural vegetables and fruits result in low glucose blood levels and elicit appropriately low insulin response. Grain-based products and sweetened foods induce elevated insulin response. The carbohydrate content of vegetables ranges from 5% to 8% and of most fruits, 8% to 14%. These foods also contain relatively high proportions of fiber. Glycemic and insulin response is low for such foods, given the low concentration of sugars and the delayed diffusion of glucose associated with fiber consumption. High glycemic food products, which are principally grain-based, range from 40% carbohydrate content and higher with substantially less fiber. Food products sweetened with refined sugars such as candies and deserts approach 80% carbohydrate content with exceedingly fiber proportions. As noted, hyperinsulinemia increases risk for type 2 diabetes, which is itself a risk factor for Mild Cognitive Impairment (Luchsinger, et al., 2007; Kodl and Sequist, 2008) and Alzheimer's disease (Arvanitakis, Wilson, Bienias, Evans, and Bennett, 2004; Ronnemaa, et al., 2008). In addition, hyperinsulinemia generates effects on neural tissue with respect to pathophysiological factors associated with neurodegeneration.

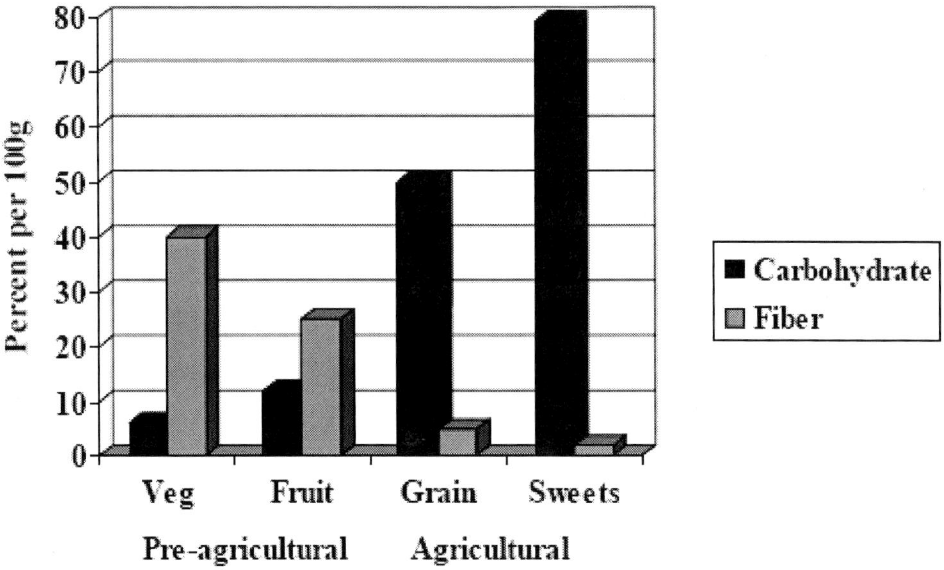

Figure 3. Carbohydrate and fiber content of common carbohydrate foods and food products.

Insulin receptors are distributed in the brain somewhat selectively with prominent representation in medial temporal lobe (hippocampus and entorhinal cortex) and in neocortex, regions that are vulnerable to Alzheimer's disease (Craft and Watson, 2004). Insulin facilitates glucose uptake in the brain, modulates neurotransmitter levels, and affects neuronal function, including signaling pertinent to memory function. At physiologically optimal levels insulin facilitates memory, as demonstrated in animal studies (Park, Seeley, Craft, and Woods, 2000) and in human studies of patients with early AD utilizing intravenous (Craft, et al., 2003) and intranasal (Reger, et al., 2008) insulin administration. Alzheimer's disease patients, who likely have insulin resistance, require higher doses to achieve modest increments in memory function.

Insulin enters the brain via a blood brain barrier transport mechanism (Banks, Jaspan, Huang and Kastin, 1997). However, chronic peripheral hyperinsulinemia leads to a gradient of central to peripheral insulin levels marked by central hypoinsulinemia (Baura, et al., 1996; Wallum, et al., 1987). Decreased brain insulin levels are associated with increased beta-amyloid peptide, a pathophysiological feature of AD and a factor that acutely impairs memory function through disruption of BDNF (brain derived neurotrophic factor) activation (Tang, Thornton, Balazs, and Cotman, 2001) and long-term potentiation (Wang, et al., 2002; Wasterman, et al., 2002). BDNF supports existing and new neuron function, especially in the hippocampus and neocortex. BDNF also is a key factor stimulating neurogenesis and is essential for long-term memory (Bekinschtein, et al., 2008). Hyperinsulinemia also upregulates free fatty acids and inflammatory cytokines, particularly in the context of obesity, and the insulin gradient has a direct effect on inflammation. In the periphery, lower levels of insulin have anti-inflammatory effects. However, at high levels, insulin is pro-inflammatory (Dandona, Alijada, and Mohanty, 2002), and these actions generate increases in a variety of inflammatory cytokines in the brain, including TNF-α (tumor necrosis factor alpha) (Fischel, et al., 2005). While TNF-α is protective against apoptosis (programmed cell death) in individuals with normal metabolism, it promotes apoptosis (Craft and Watson, 2004) in the context of insulin resistance. Accordingly, peripheral hyperinsulinemia directly increases central inflammation. In addition, higher levels of TNF-α inhibit beta-amyloid transport from the brain to the periphery where it can be cleared by the liver.

These direct actions of compensatory hyperinsulinemia generate adverse effects in brain, including increasing beta-amyloid, increasing inflammation, and reducing memory function by means of cellular mechanisms involved in learning and neural plasticity. Further, a self-reinforcing process that tends to perpetuate these effects can be established. For example, increased inflammation and increased beta-amyloid initiate a signaling cascade that increases inflammation and beta-amyloid further. Moreover, hyperinsulinemia is implicated in virtually all cardiovascular risk factors, among them increased waist circumference and obesity, hypertension, elevated triglycerides and dense, very low density lipoprotein, reduced HDL cholesterol, and the pathophysiology of type 2 diabetes (Taubes, 2007). Also, hyperinsulinemia enhances HPA axis activity and, thereby cortisol secretion (Fruehwald-Schultes, et al., 1999). Accordingly, compensatory hyperinsulinemia can be conceived as a mechanism involved in a variety of pathological processes specifically related to memory decline and AD and to other mechanisms contributing indirectly to neurodegeneration. Furthermore, the epidemiological evidence linking cardiovascular risks and disease to AD may be understood, in large part, as mediated by compensatory insulinemia, again an explanatory factor that may account for a major component of the etiology of MCI, AD, and primary vascular dementia.

Interventions in Cognitive Aging

A stage model of cognitive aging has been proposed which includes distinct phases termed *initiation* and *propagation* (Cotman, 2000). At the molecular level, the primary driving mechanisms leading to progressive loss of brain cells involve normal adaptive and protective mechanisms such as free radical activity, inflammation, and apoptosis. In the *initiation* stage early changes compromise cell function. Over time, increased injury promotes further, accelerated homeostatic responses as well as other mechanisms such as production of intracellular neurofibrillary tangles and beta amyloid-related reduction of BDNF, which contribute to neuron dysfunction (but not death) in the initiation phase. However, with chronically increased inflammation, oxidative stress, and apoptosis, neural compromise and cell death increase and the propagation phase ensues, in which neurodegenerative processes become self-reinforcing.

One might assume that Mild Cognitive Impairment corresponds roughly to the initiation phase and that Alzheimer's disease to the propagation phase. This sort of model is useful in a number of respects, but in particular because it highlights the issue of intervention timing. That is, to what point might intervention be effective, and when is it too late. Brain regions do not decline as a whole, but rather circuits associated with specific neurotransmitters degrade in the context of preserved surrounding tissue. Within the hippocampus, the preforant path (layer II of the entorhinal cortex) is susceptible to early decline with neurons transitioning from normally functioning to dysfunctional as tau neurofibriallary tangles accumulate and neurodegeneration is initiated (Morrison and Hof, 1997). Cotman proposed that cell dysfunction during initiation is potentially reversible and that intervention can be successfully invoked before the propagation phase. For example, an important inflammatory mediator, TNF-α, can initiate apopotosis but also can be protective, depending on the metabolic state of the cells. With normal metabolism, TNF-α does not induce cell death but rather signals actions that are neuroprotective. Reducing inflammatory load and normalizing the metabolic milieu in the brain (which are related processes) can serve to ameliorate function during the initiation stage. The implication is that successful therapeutic strategies invoked at or before the MCI stage might serve to salvage and reinvigorate transitional neurons and forestall the neurodegenerative process.

If we understand the diseases of civilization as diseases of hyperinsulinemia, the high prevalence of this condition and related disorders frames the question as to the basis for this state of affairs. From the point of view of preserving functional capability, health can be said to have actually declined as lifespan has increased. This has been especially true during the last 30 years during which time increasing waist circumference has been a certain marker of the decline in general health. Recent projections indicate that the percentage of overweight adults will reach 86% in 2030, with 51% of those individuals being obese (Wang, Beydoun, Liang, Caballero, and Kumanyika, 2008). It has been argued convincingly that the causes of this public health epidemic involve the deviation of contemporary lifestyle from functional adaptations consistent with our genetic endowment (Eaton, Konner, and Shostak, 1988). In a sense, the prevalence of these conditions is an index of the extent to which western societies have diverged from the environment of evolutionary adaptedness, especially as compared with more favorable environments such as that represented by Okinawa. One can make the case that with respect to stress exposure, physical activity, and diet, life in the modern world represents a substantial departure from the environment that shaped human functional attributes and the genes that underlie them. Again, dietary divergence almost certainly represents the most illustrative and most important factor, a notion exemplified by the empirical surveys of the Kitava culture (Lindeberg and Lundh, 1993).

The diet of western, industrialized societies varies substantially from pre-agricultural diets with respect to a number of factors, among them glycemic load, fatty acid composition, macronutrient composition, micronutrient density, and fiber content (Cordain, 2006). Each of these factors contributes to diseases of civilization and, thereby, to age-associated cognitive decline. We have focused on adverse effects of chronic elevation of the master hormone, insulin. While a number of dietary, physical activity, and stress factors will influence insulin sensitivity and glucose disposal, perhaps the most instructive example and the dietary factor generating the greatest effect involves glycemic load. Whereas the pre-agricultural, hunter gatherer diet consisted of 22%-40% carbohydrate, 25%-59% fat, and 19%-35% protein, the current diet in the United States is comprised, on average, of 51.8% carbohydrate, 32.8% fat, and 15.4% protein (Cordain, 2006). More importantly, the nature of the foods comprising these macronutrient categories in western cultures is quite different in specific ways that induce elevated insulin response. As examples, refined sugars comprise 18.6% of total energy, and refined grain products 20.4%, for a total of 39% of calories in the form of high glycemic load carbohydrate food products (Gerrior and Bente, 2002). Further, dairy products, which are lower in glycemic content but still highly insulinotrophic, comprise an additional

10.6% of calories (Gerrior and Bente, 2002). Accordingly, approximately 50% of daily calories are derived from foods that induce excess insulin secretion, and this highly insulinotrophic load is not much mitigated by fiber. Fiber consumption, which tends to slow glucose release and reduce insulin secretion, is just 15 g/day in the US diet compared with 42.5 g/day in primitive cultures (Cordain, 2002) and well below the recommended value (Krauss, et al., 2000). Chronic consumption of agrarian foods (Figure 3) is pervasive.

To date preventive and early intervention approaches continue to remain underdeveloped options in part because of the focus on pharmaceuticals and in part because of resistance to alteration of lifestyle habits. Nevertheless, it is important to recognize that lifestyle approaches hold promise as powerful and safe interventions because they directly influence health factors and underlying physiology that determine the course of brain aging. On the other hand, lifestyle approaches require behavior change, and this has proved to be extraordinarily difficult to accomplish in societal contexts that engender chronic stress, limited physical activity, and poor dietary choices.

While it is not possible to re-create the optimal environment in western cultures, there are changes that can be made at the individual level to avoid or circumvent adverse exposures and to induce beneficial responses. Stress reduction can be approached in terms of modifying environmental factors that maintain chronic stress and engaging in stress reducing and/or gratifying experiences that serve to lower the physiological stress response. Increasing physical activity will be helpful in maintaining lower waist circumference and weight as well as inducing other positive physiological adaptations. Strength training may be more important than aerobic exercise for aging individuals because it helps build and maintain lean body mass and bone density, which generate other health benefits including improved glucose utilization and insulin sensitivity. Physical activity can potentiate neurogenesis in the hippocampal and neocortex and increase secretion of neurotrophic factors important for neural integrity, learning, and neuroplasticity, and physical exertion causes the production of stress response proteins that work at the cellular level to mitigate free radical activity. Finally, diet can be altered to avoid high calorie, low nutrition, low fiber carbohydrate foods that potentiate insulin response and related proliferative hormones.

Conclusion

The median age of the North American population rose from 29.8 years in 1950 to 42.1 years in 1998 and is expected to continue to increase to 50 years by 2050. The number of adults aged 65 or older in the United States has increased 11-fold since 1900, and now 1 in 8 Americans is older than 65 years of age (Brookmeyer, Gray, and Kawas, 1998). In 2050, 30% of the total population will be over age 65 (Geneva, United Nations Population Division, 1998, 2003), and it is expected that the prevalence of Alzheimer's disease will increase from the current 4.5 million to 14 million cases in the United States. Furthermore, recent data concerning the prevalence of Mild Cognitive Impairment in a community sample (Petersen, et al., 2008) suggest that even these high projections may underestimate the magnitude of this public health problem. AD entails extraordinary personal cost for patients and caregivers. In addition, the annual financial cost associated with caring for patients with AD in the United

States is $148 billion to state and federal health care payers, aside from costs absorbed by the Veterans Administration, private health insurance, and families. Interventions that would delay the onset of AD by just one year would save $1.5 billion annually (Shah, Tangelos, and Petersen, 2000). Delaying onset by five years would reduce the number of cases by 50% (Alzheimer's Association, 2008). The pharmacological treatments that have become available in recent years provide time-limited, symptomatic improvement for about 50% of patients but do not address fundamental pathoetiological processes to modify disease progression (Alzheimer's Association, 2008). Given the prospects for increasing prevalence of cognitive deterioration in the elderly, prevention and early amelioration represent the optimal means of coping with this substantial public health problem.

As we have observed, aging is strongly linked to disease, and our understanding of the nature of the relationship between aging and disease is crucial in the context of guiding research intended to alter health outcomes in late life. Observation of the phenomenology of functional decline with aging suggests a distinction between the aging process and specific disease conditions associated with aging. Indeed, most aging researchers subscribe to the concept of primary and secondary aging, which assumes a distinction between these processes (Blumenthal, 2003). Primary aging refers to functional decline intrinsic to aging independent of disease and environmental effects (Shock, 1961; Busse, 1969). Secondary aging refers to deterioration resulting from disease conditions, environmental factors, and poor health practices, such as cardiovascular disorders, excess abdominal fat accumulation, sedentary lifestyle, and smoking. Under this view, disease is not intrinsic to the process of aging, although disease conditions influence aging. A corollary of the concept of primary aging is so-called normal senescence in the absence of disease, which would be relevant to our discussion of age-related neurodegenerative decline. That is, is there primary aging or normal decline of cognitive function in the absence of disease or does neurodegenerative decline occur largely in the context of disease? Is age-associated memory impairment expectable in later life? Is Alzheimer's disease inevitable for those who achieve extraordinary longevity?

Gene-environment interaction is intrinsic to aging as is evident in studies demonstrating absence or reversal of age-related conditions by environmental manipulations. Functional foods can reverse motor and cognitive deficits and age-related cellular changes in the brain (Joseph, et al., 1999), and calorie restriction eliminates commonly expected atherosclerosis in humans, even when begun in middle age (Fontana, Meyer, Klein, and Holloszy, 2004). Health factors (functional status and disease conditions) can be used as an index of the gene-environment interaction so that health maintenance efforts become a matter of modulating environmental factors to bias this interaction toward slowing the rate of aging. Thus, from the point of view of disease prevention, it is prudent to control and mitigate environmental exposures that will accelerate aging and disease promoting processes.

Whether one finds the primary-secondary aging distinction useful, it is apparent that chronic disease conditions influence brain health and modulate risk for neurodegeneration. Contemporary industrialized cultures provide safeguards and interventions that increase longevity while simultaneously fostering overall adaptation that tends to promote and/or maintain disease and neurodegeneration. The apparent optimization of the gene-environment interaction represented by the Okinawan cohort was to a major extent imposed by poverty and isolation from industrialization. In a sense, this observation provides further evidence that the affluence and many of the attendant lifestyle changes in developed cultures generate conditions that are less than optimal from the point of view of health span and preservation of cognition in late life. To a large extent, the interventions aimed at stress control, maintaining physical activity, and dietary modification represent approaches designed to avoid and compensate for aspects of the culture that adversely influence organism adaptations and increase risk for disease and neurodegeneration. While it would be extraordinarily difficult in the short term to alter the structure of developed societies in ways that would decrease aging risks, it is feasible to alter behavior and the environment at the individual level for optimal preservation of function into old age. And, to the extent that there are empirical demonstrations of benefit from these approaches, we can work toward the ultimate adoption of cultural changes that will provide for enjoyment of the advantages of the modern world but also preserve health and cognition throughout the lifespan.

References

Alzheimer's Association. (2008). *2008 Alzheimer's disease facts and figures*. Chicago, IL: Alzheimer's Association.

Anderson-Ranberg, K., Schroll, M., and Jeune, B. (2001). Healthy centenarians do not exist, but autonomous centenarians do: A population-based study of morbidity among Danish centenarians. *Journal of the American Geriatrics Society, 49*, 900-908.

Applegate, W. B., Pressel, S., Wittes, J., Luhr, J., Shekelle, R. B., Camel, G. H., et al. (1994). Impact of the treatment of isolated systolic hypertension on behavioral variables. *Archives of Internal Medicine, 154*, 2154-2160.

Alves de Moraes, S., Szklo, M., Knopman, D., and Sato, R. (2002). The relationship between temporal changes in blood pressure and changes in cognitive function: Atherosclerosis risk in communities (ARIC) study. *Preventive Medicine, 35*, 258-263.

Arvanitakis, Z., Wilson, R. S., Bienias, J. L.., Evans, D. A., and Bennett, D. (2004). Diabetes mellitus and risk of Alzheimer disease and decline in cognitive function. *Archives of Neurology, 61*, 661-666.

Backman, L., Jones, S., Berger, A. K., Laukka, E. J., and Small, B. J. (2005). Cognitive impairment in preclinical Alzheimer's disease: A meta-analysis. *Neuropsychology, 19*, 520-531.

Ballard, C., O'Brien, J., Barber, B., Scheltens, P., Shaw, F., McKeith, I., et al. (2000). Neurocardiovascular instability, hypotensive episodes, and MRI lesions in neurodegenerative dementia. *Annals of the New York Academy of Sciences, 903*, 442-445.

Banks, W. A., Jaspan, J. B., Huang, W., and Kastin A. J. (1997). Transport of insulin across the blood-brain barrier: Saturability at euglycemic doses of insulin. *Peptides, 18,* 1421-1429.

Baura, G. D., Foster, D. M., Kaiyala, K., Porte, D., Kahn, S. E., and Schwartz, M. W. (1996). Insulin transport from plasma into the central nervous system is inhibited by dexamethasone in dogs. *Diabetes, 45*, 86-90.

Bekinschtein, P., Cammarota, M., Katche, C., Slipczuk, L., Rossato, J. I., Goldin, A., et al. (2008). BDNF is essential to promote persistence of long-term memory storage. *Proceedings of the National Academy of Sciences*, *105*, 2711-2716.

Blumenthal, H.T. (2003). The aging-disease dichotomy: True or false? *Journal of Gerontology*, *58A*, 138-145.

Bowen, J., Teri L., Kukull, W., McCormick, W., McCurry, S. M., and Larson, E. B. (1997). Progression to dementia in patients with isolated memory loss. *Lancet*, 349, 763-765.

Brady, C. B., Spiro, A., and Gaziano, J. M. (2005). Effects of age and hypertension status on cognition: The Veterans Affairs Normative Aging study. *Neuropsychology*.19, 770-777.

Breteler, M. M. (2000). Vascular risk factors for Alzheimer's disease: An epidemiologic perspective. *Neurobiology of Aging*, *21*, 153-160.

Brookmeyer, R., Gray, S., and Kawas, C. (1998). Projections of Alzheimer's disease in the United States and the public health impact of delaying disease onset. *American Journal of Public Health*, 88, 1337-1342.

Brown, E. S., Rush, J., and McEwen, B. S. (1999). Hippocampal remodeling and damage by corticosteroids: Implications for mood disorders. *Neuropsychopharmacology*, *21*, 474-484.

Busse, E. W. (1969). Theories of aging. In E. W. Busse and E. Pfeiffer (Eds.), *Behavior and adaptation in adult life* (p 11-32). Boston: Little Brown.

Centers for Disease Control and Prevention (CDC). (2004). *National Center for Health Statistics (NCHS)*. National Health and Nutrition Examination Survey Data. Hyattsville, MD: US Department of Health and Human Services, Centers for Disease Control and Prevention.

Chertkow, H., Massoud, F., Nasreddine, Z., Belleville, S., Joanette, Y., Bocti, C., et al. (2008). Diagnosis and treatment of dementia: 3. Mild cognitive impairment and cognitive impairment without dementia. *Canadian Medical Association Journal, 178*(10), 1273-1285.

Coppola, C. L., Grandin, T., and Enns, R. M. (2006). Human interaction and cortisol: Can human contact reduce stress for shelter dogs? *Physiology and Behavior*, *87*, 537-541.

Cordain, L. (2002). The nutritional characteristics of a contemporary diet based upon Paleolithic food groups. *Journal of the American Nutraceutical Association*, *5*, 15-24.

Cordain L. (2006). Implications of Plio-Pleistocene Hominin Diets for Modern Humans. In : P Ungar (Ed.), *Early hominin diets: The known, the unknown, and the unknowable.*, pp 363-383, Oxford University Press, Oxford.

Cotman, C. W. (2000). Homeostatic processes in brain aging: The role of apoptosis, inflammation, and oxidative stress in regulating healthy neural circuitry in the aging brain. In P Stern, L Carstensen (Eds.), *National Research Council, The aging mind: Opportunities in cognitive research.* Washington DC: National Academy Press.

Craft, S. (2005). Insulin resistance syndrome and Alzheimer's disease: Age- and obesity-related effects on memory, amyloid, and inflammation. *Neurobiology of Aging*, *26S*, S65-S69.

Craft, S., Asthana, S., Cook, D. G., Bader, L. D., Cherrier, M., Purganan, K., et al. (2003). Insulin dose-response effects on memory and plasma amyloid precursor protein in

Alzheimer's disease: Interactions with apolipoprotein E genotype. *Psychoneuroendocrinology, 28*, 809-822.

Craft, C. and Watson, G. S. (2004). Insulin and neurodegenerative disease: Shared and specific mechanisms. *Lancet Neurology, 3*, 169-178.

Crook, T. H., Bartus, R. T., Ferris, S. H., Whitehouse, P., Cohen, G. D., and Gershon, S. (1986). Age-associated memory impairment: Proposed diagnostic criteria and measures of clinical change. *Developmental Neuropsychology, 3*, 261-276.

Dandona, P., Aljada, A., and Mohanty, P. (2002). The anti-inflammatory and potential anti-atherogenic effect of insulin: A new paradigm. *Diabetologia, 45*, 924-930.Davis, K. L., Davis, B. M., Greenwald, B. S., Mohs, R. C., Mathe, A. A., Johns, C. A., and Horvath TB (1986). Cortisol and Alzheimer's disease I: Basal studies. *American Journal of Psychiatry, 143*, 300-305.

Department of Health and Human Services, Centers for Disease Control and Prevention. (2004). *National Health and Nutrition Examination Survey Data.* Hyattsville, MD: US Department of Health and Human Services, Centers for Disease Control and Prevention

de Leon, M., Golomb, J., George, A. E, Convit, A., Tarshish, C. Y., McRae, T., et al. (1993). The radiologic prediction of Alzheimer disease: The atrophic hippocampal formation. *Amerian Journal of Neuroradiology, 14*, 897-906.

de Leon, M. J., Convit, A., Wolf, O. T., Tarshish, C. Y., DeSanti, S., Rusinek, H., et al. (2001). Prediction of cognitive decline in normal elderly subjects with 2-[^{18}F]fluoro-2-deoxy-d-gucose/positron-emission tomography (FDG/PET). *Proceedings of the National Academy of Sciences, 98*, 10966-10971.

Ditzen, B., Schmidt, S., Strauss, B., Nater, R. M., Ehlert, U., and Heinrichs, M. (2008). Adult attachment and social support interact to reduce psychological but no cortisol responses to stress. *Journal of Psychosomatic Research, 64*, 479-486.

Dufouil, C., Chalmers, J., Coskun, O., Besançon, V., Bousser, M. G., Guillon, P., et al. (2005). Effects of blood pressure lowering on cerebral white matter hyperintensities in patients with stroke: The PROGRESS magnetic resonance imaging substudy. *Circulation. 112*,1644-1650.

Eaton, S. B., Konner, M., and Shostak, M. (1988). Stone agers in the fast lane: Chronic degenerative diseases in evolutionary perspective. *American Journal of Medicine, 84*, 739-749.

Ebly, E. M., Hogan, D. B., and Parhad, I. M. (1995). Cognitive impairment in the nondemented elderly. Results from the Canadian Study of Health and Aging. *Archives of Neurology, 52*, 612-619.

Elias, P. K, Elias, M. F., D'Agostino, R. B., Cupples, L. A., Wilson, P. W., Silbershatz, H., et al. (1997). NIDDM and blood pressure as risk factors for poor cognitive performance. *Diabetes Care, 20*, 1388-1395

Elias, M. F., Elias, P. K., Sullivan, L. M., Wolf, P. A., and D'Agostino, R. B. (2003). Lower cognitive function in the presence of obesity and hypertension: The Framingham heart study. *International Journal of Obesity, 27*, 260-268.

Farkas, E., DeVos, R. A., Steur, E. N., and Luiten, P. G. (2000). Are Alzheimer's disease, hypertension, and cerebrocapillary damage related? *Neurobiology of Aging, 21*, 235-243.

Fishel, M. A., Watson, G. S., Montine, T. J., Wang, Q., Greene, P. S., Kulstad, J. J., et al., (2005). Hyperinsulinemia provokes synchronous increases in central inflammation and ß-amyloid in normal adults. *Archives of Neurology*, *62*, 1539-1544.

Flicker, C., Ferris, S. H, and Reisberg, B. (1991). Mild cognitive impairment in the elderly: Predictors of dementia. *Neurology, 41*, 1006-1009.

Fontana, L., Meyer, T. E., Klein, S., and Holloszy, J. O. (2004). Long-term calorie restriction is highly effective in reducing the risk of atherosclerosis in humans. *Proceedings of the National Academy of Sciences*, *101*, 6659-6663.

Fratiglioni, L., Wang, H., Ericsson, K., Maytan, M., and Winblad, B. (2000). Influence of social network on occurrence of dementia: A community-based longitudinal study. *Lancet*, *355*, 1315-1319.

Fruehwald-Schultes, B., Kern, W., Bong, W., Wellhoener, P., Kerner, W., Born, J., et al. (1999). Supraphysiological hyperinsulinemia acutely increases hypothalamic-pituitary-adrenal secretory activity in humans. *Journal of Clinical Endocrinology and Metabolism*, *84*, 3041-3046.

Gage, F. H., Kempermann, G., Palmer, T. D., Peterson, D. A., and Ray, J. (1998). Multipotent progenitor cells in the adult dentate gyrus. *J. Neurobiol*, *36*, 249-266.

Geneva, United Nations, Population Division, (1998; 2003). *Ageing and The Oldest Old*, Department of Economics and Social Affairs.

Gerrier, S. and Bente, L. (2002). *Nutrient content of the U.S. food supply, 1909-1999: A summary report.* United States Department of Agriculture, Center for Nutrition Policy and Promotion. Home Economics Report No. 55.

Goff, D. C., Zaccaro, D. J., Hafner, S. M., and Saad, M. F . (2003). Insulin sensitivity and the risk of incident hypertension: Insights from the Insulin Resistance Atherosclerosis Study. *Diabetes Care*, *26*, 805-811.

Goldman, W. P, and Morris, J. C. (2001). Evidence that age-associated memory impairment is not a normal variant of aging. *Alzheimer Disease and Associated Disorders,15*:72-79.

Gould, E., Reeves, A. J., Graziano, M. S., and Gross, C. G. (1999). Neurogenesis in the neocortex of adult primates. *Science*, *286*, 548-552.

Green, K. N, Billings, L. M, Roozendaal, B., McGaugh, J. L, and LaFerla, F. M. (2006). Glucocorticoids increase amyloid-ß and tau pathology in a mouse model of Alzhiemer's disease. *Journal of Neuroscience, 30*, 9047-56.

Heinrichs, M., Baumgarten, T., Kirschbaum, C., and Ehlert, U. (2003). Social support and oxytocin interact to suppress cortisol and subjective responses to psychosocial stress. *Biological Psychiatry*, *54*, 1389-1398.

Hershey, T., Perantie, D. C., Warren, S. L., Zimmerman, E. C., Sadler, M., and White, N. H. (2005). Frequency and timing of severe hypoglycemia affets spatial memory in children with type 1 diabetes. *Diabetes Care*, *28*, 2372-2377.

Hofman, A., Ott, A., Breteler, M. M., Bots, M. L., Slooter, A. J., van Harskamp, F., et al. (1997). Atherosclerosis, apolipoprotein E, and prevalence of dementia and Alzheimer's disease in the Rotterdam study. *Lancet*, *349*, 151-154.

Holtzman, D. M., Bales, K. R., Tenkova, T., Fagan, A. M., Parsadanian, M., Sartorius, L. J., et al. (2000). Apolipoprotein E isoform-dependent amyloid deposition and neuritic degeneration in a mouse model of Alzheimer's disease. *Proceedings of the National Academy of Sciences, 97*, 2892-2897.

Joseph, J. A., Shukitt-Hale, B., Denisova, N. A., Bielinski, D., Martin A., McEwen, J. J., et al. (1999). Reversals of age-related declines in neuronal signal transduction, cognitive and motor behavioral deficits with blueberry, spinach or strawberry dietary supplementation. *Journal of Neuroscience, 19,* 8114-8121.

Kalaria, R. N. (2000). The role of cerebral ischemia in Alzheimer's disease. *Neurobiology of Aging, 21*, 321-330.

Kodl, C. T., and Sequist, E. R. (2008). Cognitive dysfunction and diabetes mellitus. *Endocrine Reviews, 29*, 494-511.

Kokmen, E., Beard, M. C., O'Brien, P. C., and Kurland, L. T. (1996). Epidemiology of dementia in Rochester, Minnesota. *Mayo Clinic Proceedings, 71*, 275-282.

Krauss, R. M., Eckel, R. H., Howard, B., Appel, L. J., Daniels, S. K., Deckelbaum, R. J., et al. (2000). AHA dietary guidelines revision 2000: A statement for healthcare professionals from the nutrition committee of the American Heart Association. *Circulation, 102*, 2284-2299.

Krikorian, R. (1996). Independence of verbal and spatial paired associate learning. *Brain and Cognition, 32*, 219-223.

Krikorian, R. (2006). Cognitive changes in perimenopause. In M Gass, J Liu (Eds.), *Management of the perimenopause*. New York: McGraw-Hill.

La Rue, A. (1992). *Aging and neuropsychological assessment*. New York: Plenum Press.

Lester, M. L., Thatcher, R. W., and Monroe-Lord, L. (1982). Refined carbohydrate intake, hair cadmium levels and cognitive functioning in children. *Nutrition and Behavior, 1*, 1-14.

Lindeberg, S., Eliasson, M., Lindahl, B., and Ahren, B. (1999). Low serum insulin in traditional Pacific Islanders: The Kitava Study. *Metabolism, 48*, 1216-1219.

Lindeberg, S., and Lundh, B. (1993). Apparent absence of stroke and ischaemic heart disease in a traditional Melanesian island: A clinical study in Kitava. *Journal of Internal Medicine, 233*, 269-275.

Luchsinger, J. A., Reitz, C., Patel, B., Tang, M., Manly, J. J., and Mayeux, R. (2007). Relation of diabetes to Mild Cognitive Impairment. *Archives of Neurology, 64*, 570-575.

Lui, Q., Zerbinatti, C.V., Zhang, J., Hoe, H., Wang, B., Cole, S. L.,et al. (2007). Amyloid precursor protein regulates brain apolipoprotein E and cholesterol metabolism through lipoprotein receptor LRP1. *Neuron, 56*, 66-78.

Lupien, S. J., de Leon, M., de Santi, S., Convit, A., Tarshish, C., Nair, N. P., et al. (1998). Cortisol levels during human aging predict hippocampal atrophy and memory deficits. *Nature Neuroscience, 1*, 69-73.

Lupien, S. J., Nair, N. P., Briere, S., Maheu, F., Tu, M. T., Lemay, M., et al.(1999). Increased cortisol levels and impaired cognition in human aging. *Reviews in the Neurosciences, 10*, 117-139.

Lupien, S. J., Wilkinson, C. W., Briere, S., Kin, N. M., Meaney, M. J., and Nair, N. P. (2002). Acute modulation of aged human memory by pharmacological manipulation of glucocorticoids. *Journal of Clinical Endocrinology and Metabolism, 87*, 3798-3807.

Lupien, S. J., Fiocco, A., Wan, N., Maheu, F., Lord, C., Schramek, T., et al. (2005). Stress hormones and human memory function across the lifespan. *Psychoneuroendocrinology, 30*, 225-242.

Madden, D. J., and Blumenthal, J. A. (1998). Interaction of hypertension and age in visual selective attention performance. *Health Psychol*olgy, *17*, 76-83.

Masoro, E. J. (2006). Are age-associated diseases an integral part of aging? In E. J. Masoro and S. Austad S (Eds.) *Handbook of the biology of aging, sixth edition*. Academic Press: Boston.

McEwen, B. S., de Leon, M., Lupien, S. J., and Meaney, M. J. (1999). Corticosteroids, the aging brain and cognition. *Trends in Endocrinology and Metabolism, 10*, 92-96.

Morrison, J. H., and Jof, P. R. (1997). Life and death of neurons in the aging brain. *Science, 278*, 412-419.

Muldoon, M. F., Waldstein, S. R., Ryan, C. M., Jennings, J. R., Polefrone, J. M., Shapiro, A. P., et al. (2002). Effects of six anti-hypertensive medications on cognitive performance. *Journal of Hypertension, 20*, 1643-1652.

Murray, M. D., Lane, K. A., Gao, S., Evans, R. M., Unverzagt, F. W., Hall, K. S., et al. (2002-). Preservation of cognitive function with antihypertensive medications: A longitudinal analysis of a community-based sample of African Americans. *Archives of Internal Medicine, 162*, 2090-2096.

Nagy, Z., Esiri, M. M., Hindley, N. J., Joachim, C., Morris, J. H., King, E. M., et al. (1998). Accuracy of clinical operational diagnostic criteria for Alzheimer's disease in relation to different pathological diagnostic protocols. *Dementia and Geriatric Cognitive Disorders, 9*, 219-26.

Neilsen, H., Lolk, A., and Kragh-Sorensen, P. (1998). Age-associated memory impairment – pathological memory decline or normal aging? *Scandavian Journal of Psychology, 39*, 33-37.

Ogura, C., Nakamoto, H., Uema, T., Yamamoto, K., Yonemori, T., Yoshimura, T., et al. (1995). Prevalence of senile dementia in Okinawa, Japan. *International Journal of Epidemiology, 24*, 373-380.

Park, C. R., Seeley, R. J., Craft, S., and Woods, S. C. (2000). Intracerebroventricular insulin enhances memory in a passive-avoidance task. *Physiology and Behavior, 68*, 509-514.

Pasquier, F., Leya, D., and Scheltens, P. (1998). The influence of coincidental vascular pathology on symptomatology and course of Alzheimer's disease. *Journal of Neural Transmission, 54*, 117-127.

Perls, T. (2004). Dementia-free centenarians. *Experimental Gerontology, 39*, 1587-1593.

Petersen, R. C., Roberts, R., Knopman, D. S., Geda, Y., Pankratz, V., Boeve, B. F., et al. (2008, July). *The Mayo Clinic study of aging: Incidence of mild cognitive impairment.* Paper presented at the International Conference on Alzheimer's Disease, Chicago..

Petersen, R. C., Smith, G. E., Ivnik, R. J., Kokmen, E., Tangalos, E. G. (1994). Memory function in very early Alzheimer's disease. *Neurology, 44*, 867-872.

Petersen, R. C., Smith, G. E,. Waring, S. C., Ivnik, R. J., Tangalos, E. G., and Kokmen, E. (1999). Mild Cognitive Impairment: Clinical characterization and outcome. *Archives of Neurology, 56*, 303-308.

Petersen, R. C., Doody, R., Kurz, A., Mohs, R. C., Morris, J. C., Rabins, P. V., et al. (2001). Current Concepts in Mild Cognitive Impairment. *Archives of Neurology, 58*, 1985-1992.

Plassman, B. L., Langa, K. M., Fisher, G. G., Heeringa, S. G., Weir, D. R., Ofstedal, M. B., et al. (2007). Prevalence of dementia in the United States: The aging, demographics, and memory study. *Neuroepidemiology, 29*, 125-132.

Porter, N. M, and Landfield, P. W (1998). Stress hormones and brain aging: adding injury to insult? *Nature Neuroscience, 1*, 3-4.

Raz, N., Rodrigue, K. M, and Acher, J. D. (2003). Hypertension and the brain: Vulnerability of the prefrontal regions and executive functions. *Behavioral Neuroscience., 117*, 1169-1180.

Reger, M., Watson, G. S., Cholerton, B., Baker, L., Asthana, S., Plymate, S., et al. (2004). Cortisol infusion attenuates insulin's facilitation of verbal memory in patients with Alzheimer's disease. *Neurobiology of Aging, 25 (S2)*, 168.

Reger, M. A., Watson, G. S., Green, P. S., Wilkinson, C. W., Baker, L. D., Cholerton, B., et al. (2008). Intranasal insulin improves cognition and modulates ß-amyloid in early AD. *Neurology, 70*, 440-448.

Reaven, G. M. (1988). Role of insulin resistance in human disease. *Diabetes, 37*, 1495-1607.

Reaven, G. M. (1994). Syndrome X: 6 years later. *Journal of Internal Medicine, 236*, 12.-22.

Resnick, H., Jones, K., Ruotolo, G., Jain, A., Henderson, J, Lu, W. , et al. (2003). Insulin resistance, the metabolic syndrome and risk of incident cardiovascular disease in nondiabetic American Indians, *Diabetes Care, 26*, 861-867.

Rönnemaa, E., Zethelius, B., Sundelöf, J., Sundström, J., Degerman-Gunnarsson, M., Berne, C., et al. (2008). Impaired insulin secretion increases the risk of Alzheimer disease. *Neurology, 71,* 1065-1071.

Rosal, M. C., King, J. A., Ma, Y., and Reed, G. W. (2004). Stress, social support, and cortisol: Inverse associations. *Behavioral Medicine, 30*, 11-21.

Rowe, J. W., and Kahn, R.W. (1998). *Successful aging*. New York: Pantheon Books.

Swanwick, G. R., Kirby, M., Bruce, I., Buggy, F., Coen, R. F., Coakley, D., et al. (1998). Hypothalamic-pituitary-adrenal axis dysfunction in Alzheimer's disease: Lack of association between longitudinal and cross-sectional findings. *American Journal of Psychiatry, 155*, 286-289.

Scuteri, A., Naijar, S. S., Muller, D. C., Andres, R., Hougaku, H., Metter, E. J., et al. (2004). Metabolic syndrome amplifies the age-associated increases in vascular thickness and stiffness. *Journal of the American College of Cardiology, 43*, 1388-1395.

Seeman, T. E., and McEwen, B. S. (1996). Impact of social environmental characteristics on endocrine regulation. *Psychosomatic Medicine, 58*, 459-471.

Shah, T., Tangalos, E. G, and Petersen, R. C (2000). Mild Cognitive Impairment: When is it a precursor to Alzheimer's disease. *Geriatrics, 55*, 62-68.

Shaw, D. I., Hall, W. L., and Williams, C.M. (2005). Metabolic syndrome: What is it and what are the implications? *Proceedings of the Nutrition Society, 64*, 349-357.

Shock, N. (1961). Physiological aspects of aging. *Annual Review of Physiology, 23*, 97-122.

Skoog, I., and Gustafson, D. (2003). Hypertension, hypertension-clustering factors and Alzheimer's disease. *Neurological Research, 25,* 675-680.

Spaan, P. E., Raaijmakers, J. G., and Jonder, C. (2005). Early assessment of dementia: The contribution of different memory components. *Neuropsychology*, *19*, 629-640.

Squire, L. R., Stark, C.E.L., and Clark, R. E. (2004). The medial temporal lobe. *Annual Review of Neuroscience*, *27*, 279-306.

Starkman, M. N., Giordani, B., Gebarski, S., Berent, S., Schork, M. A., and Schteingart, D. E. (2000). Decrease in cortisol reverses human hippocampal atrophy following treatment of Cushing's disease. *Biological Psychiatry*, *46*, 1595-1602.

Starkman, M. N., Giordani, B., Gebarski, S. S., and Schteingart, D. E. (2003). Improvement in learning associated with increase in hippocampal formation volume. *Biological Psychiatry*, *53*, 233-238.

Swan, F. E., Carmelli, D., and La Rue, A. (1998). Systolic blood pressure tracking over 25 to 30 years and cognitive performance in older adults. *Stroke*, *29*, 2334-2340.

Swanwick, G. R, Kirby, M., Bruce, I., Buggy, F., Coen, R.F., Coakley, D., et al. (1998). Hypothalamic-pituitary-adrenal axis dysfunction in Alzheimer's disease: Lack of association between longitudinal and cross-sectional findings. *American Journal of Psychiatry, 155*, 286-289.

Taubes, G. (2007). *Good calories, bad calories.* New York: Knopf.

Tong, L., Thornton, P. L., Balazs, R., and Cotman, C.W. (2001). Beta-amyloid-(l-42) impairs activity-dependent cAMP-response element-binding protein signaling in neurons at concentrations in which cell survival is not compromised. *Journal of Biological Chemistry*, *276*, 17301-17306.

Wang, Y, Beydoun, M. A., Liang, L., Caballero, B., and Kumanyika, S. K. (2008). Will all Americans become overweight or obese? Estimating the progression and cost of the US obesity epidemic. *Obesity*, *16*, 2323-2330.

Wang, H.W., Pasternak, J. F., Kuo, H., Ristic, H., Lambert, M. P., Chromy, B., et al. (2002). Soluble oligomers of beta amyloid (l-42) inhibit long-term potentiation but not long-term depression in rat dentate gyrus. *Brain Research*, *924*, 133-140.

Wallum, B. J., Taborsky, G. J., Porte, D., Figlewicz, D. P., Jacobseon, L., Beard, J. C., et al. (1987). Cerebrospinal fluid insulin levels increase during intravenous insulin infusions in man. *Journal of Clinical Endocrinology and Metabolism*, *64*, 190-194.

Westerman, M. A., Cooper-Blacketer, S. D., Mariash, A., Kotilinek, S. L., Dawarabayashi, T., Younkin, L. H., et al. (2002). The relationship between Abeta and memory in the Tg2576 mouse model of Alzheimer's disease. *Journal of Neuroscience*, *22*, 1858-1867.

Willcox, B. J., Willcox, D.C., He, Q., Curb, J. D., and Suzuki M. (2006). Siblings of Okinawan centenarians exhibit lifelong mortality advantages. *Journals of Gerontology: Series A, Biological Sciences and Medical Sciences*, *61*, 345-354.

Willcox, D. C., Willcox, B. J., Todoriki, J, Curb J. D., and Suzuki, M. (2006). Caloric restriction and human longevity: What can we learn from the Okinawans? *Biogerontology*, *7*, 173-177.

Wilson, R. S., Barnes, L. L., Bennett, D. A., Li, Y., Bienias, J. L., Mendes,C. F., et al. (2005). Proneness to psychological distress and risk of Alzheimer's disease in a biracial community. *Neurology*, *64*, 380-382.

Zerbinatti, C.V., and Bu, G. (2005). LRP and Alzheimer's disease. *Reviews in the Neurosciences*, *16*, 123-135.

In: New Directions in Aging Research
Editor: Ruby R. Brougham, pp. 25-37
ISBN 978-1-60741-976-1
© 2009 Nova Science Publishers, Inc.

Chapter 2

Adult BMI and Dimensions of Psychological Well-Being: The Role of Gender

Jamila Bookwala and Jenny Boyar
Department of Psychology, Lafayette College, Easton, PA, USA

Abstract

We used data from the National Survey of Midlife Development in the United States to compare 3,322 adult men and women in normal-weight, overweight, and obese categories on psychological well-being. We found significant differences by body weight on specific dimensions of psychological well-being after controlling for socio-demographic variables, such that obese individuals scored lower than their normal and overweight counterparts.

We also found that gender moderates the link between body weight and psychological well-being. Overweight or obese women scored significantly worse on psychological well-being than normal-weight women whereas men's psychological well-being did not vary by body weight. Interestingly, normal-weight women enjoyed better psychological well-being than their male peers; obese women scored significantly worse on psychological well-being, however, than obese men. This overall pattern of results was replicated even after controlling for perceived weight. These findings are discussed in relation to research on stigma theory and gender-differentiated cultural norms regarding weight.

Keywords: Gender; BMI; psychological well-being

Introduction

Obesity has emerged as one of the most serious health concerns in the United States (Flegal, Carroll, Ogden, and Johnson, 2002; Friedman and Brownell, 1995; Ogden, et al., 2006). Flegal, et al. (2002)report that more than half the US population can be categorized as overweight (characterized by a body mass index [BMI] of 25 or higher) or obese (characterized by a BMI of 30 or higher). In terms of obesity alone, Ogden et al. (2006) reported that 31.1% of adult men and 33.2% of adult women in the US were obese in 2005. Although trends over a six-year period (1999-2004) indicate that increases in the prevalence of obesity among adult women have leveled off (but remain high), Ogden, et al. (2006) report that the proportion of men that are obese has increased by 3.6% over the same time period.

In contrast with the strong link between overweight/obesity and poorer physical well-being (National Heart, Lung, and Blood Institute [NHLBI], 1998; World Health Organization, 2002), the link between these weight categories and psychological well-being is less clear-cut (Friedman and Brownell, 1995; NHLBI, 1998), with empirical studies showing inconsistent relationships between BMI and poor mental health. Early studies found little or no association between obesity and negative psychological outcomes (see Friedman and Brownell, 1995; O'Neil and Jarrell, 1992; Wadden and Stunkard, 1993) whereas more recent studies have reported an association between overweight/obesity and poorer psychological well-being (Carr and Friedman, 2006; Friedman, Reichmann, Constanzo, and Musante, 2002; Friedman, et al., 2005; Simon, et al., 2006).

Studies conducted on convenience samples of treatment-seeking obese individuals also have found gender differences, such that obese women were more likely to exhibit depressive symptoms than were obese men (e.g., Linde, et al., 2004; Stunkard, Faith, and Allison,, 2003). A recent study using a probability-based sample also supports a similar moderating role of gender in the link between obesity and depressive mood (Heo, Pietrobelli, Fontaine, Sirey, and Faith,., 2006). The present study aimed to further current understanding in this area by examining the moderating role of gender in the relationship between BMI and different domains of psychological well-being. Our study uses a large probability-based national sample of adults who participated in the National Survey of Midlife Development in the United States (Brim, et al., 2003). We hypothesized that 1) overweight and obese respondents will experience poorer psychological well-being compared to normal-weight respondents and; 2) overweight and obese women will have poorer psychological well-being compared to their female counterparts of normal weight and to their male counterparts regardless of their BMI. It should be noted that existing studies on BMI and psychological well-being have not accounted for the likely contribution of perceived weight (viewing oneself to be of normal or excessive weight) to psychological well-being even though a reliable relationship has been found between body image and psychological well-being (e.g., Davison and McCabe, 2005; Franzoi and Herzog, 1986; McKinley, 1999; Weaver and Byers, 2006). Because we contend that it is important for studies on the link between BMI to parse the effects of BMI on psychological well-being from those of body image (or perceived weight), we examined differences in psychological well-being as a function of BMI both with and without perceived weight as a statistical covariate. In this way, we are able to provide a clearer understanding of the links among gender, BMI, and dimensions of psychological well-being.

Method

Sample

The sample for this study was drawn from adults participating in the National Survey of Midlife Development in the United States (MIDUS; Brim, et al., 2003). MIDUS was designed to assess a wide variety of patterns, predictors, and outcomes related to physical health, psychological well-being, and social responsibility during the adulthood years. It assessed these variables in 1995-1996 in a nationally representative sample of individuals between the ages of 25 and 74 years using telephone and mail questionnaires. The present study sample (N=3,322) included MIDUS respondents who had a normal or higher body mass index (BMI $\geq$ 18.5), and had complete data on all study variables. On average, the sample was 47.2 years of age (range=25-74; *SD*=13.2); 51.2% (N=1,759) of the respondents were male, 86.1% (N=2,955) described themselves to be White, 62.7% (N=2,162) had at least some college education, and almost 64% (N=2,193) were married.

Measures

Sociodemographic Variables. Data on respondents' gender, age, race, education, and marital status were used from MIDUS. For the data analyses, we dichotomized race (White vs. Other) and marital status (not married vs. married).

Body Mass Index: Participants provided data on their weight (in pounds) and height (in inches). In order to compute BMI, respondents' weight was converted into kilograms (weight in pounds X 0.4536) and their height was converted into meters (height in inches X 0.0254). Finally, BMI was calculated by taking respondents' weight in kilograms and dividing by height in meters-squared. Using the guidelines recommended by the National Heart, Lung, and Blood Institute (1998), BMI was trichotomized to form three BMI groups – respondents with a BMI of 18.5 but less than 25 were categorized as normal-weight (n = 1335); those with a BMI of $\geq$ 25 but less than 30 were categorized as overweight (n = 1263) and; those with a BMI of $\geq$ 30 were categorized as obese (n = 724).

Psychological Well-being. Six widely accepted indicators of psychological well-being, as defined by Ryff (1989), were included in MIDUS (3 items for each indicator): positive relations with others (e.g., "maintaining close relationships has been difficult and frustrating for me"), self-acceptance (e.g., "I like most parts of my personality"), autonomy ("I tend to be influenced by people with strong opinions"), personal growth (e.g., "For me, life has been a continual process of learning, changing, and growth"), environmental mastery (e.g., "The demands of everyday life often get me down"), and purpose in life (e.g., "Some people wander aimlessly through life, but I am not one of them"). Responses were made on a 7-point scale ranging from 1=strongly agree to 7=strongly disagree. Positive items were reverse coded so that higher scores represented greater levels of psychological well-being; items for each subscale were summed to yield a total score. Ryff's (1989) subscales assessing psychological well-being were generated from multiple theoretical accounts of positive functioning. The subset of items for each subscale included in the MIDUS was drawn from the original scales. These shortened scales correlated from .70 to .89 with the 20-item parent scales (Ryff and Keyes, 1995). Cronbach's alpha values were computed for these three-item measures of psychological well-being after adjusting for length of the 3-item measures using Nunnally's (1978) correction formula for computing scale reliability. When the 3-item measures were increased by a factor of 7 (n=21, to approximate the original 20-item subscales), internal consistency estimates for the six measures of psychological well-being ranged from .78 to .93.

Perceived Weight. MIDUS included a single-item measure of respondents' perceived weight, which we used as an indicator of body image. Respondents were asked to describe themselves on a 5-point scale ranging from very underweight to about the right weight to very overweight. Perceived weight was significantly correlated with BMI (r=.65), with higher BMI related to the perception of being overweight.

Results

Goal 1: BMI – Psychological Well-Being Link

In order to determine the association between BMI and psychological well-being in this sample of adults, we performed a one-way multivariate analysis of covariance (MANCOVA). Participants' age, gender, race, education, and marital status were included as covariates. The MANCOVA yielded a significant multivariate main effect of BMI group on the set of psychological well-being indicators (F[12, 6620]=3.83, p<.001). Significant univariate effects of BMI group were obtained for five of the six subscales: positive relations with others (F[2,3314]=3.54, $p < .05$), self-acceptance (F[2,3314]=3.73, $p < .05$), personal growth (F[2,3314]=13.71, $p < .001$), environmental mastery (F[2,3314]=4.84, $p < .01$), and purpose in life (F[2,3314]=3.87, $p < .05$).

In order to determine the role of BMI on psychological well-being net of perceived weight (our indicator of body image), we re-ran the above MANCOVA using perceived weight as an additional statistical covariate. Even after controlling for the effects of perceived weight emerged as a significant covariate, we obtained a significant multivariate main effect for BMI group (F[12,6444]=2.86, $p < .05$). The univariate effects remained significant for personal growth (F[2,3226]=4.44, $p < .05$) and purpose in life (F[2,3226]=8.07, $p < .01$) after controlling for the effects of perceived weight; no other univariate effects reached statistical significance.

LSD post hoc comparisons for the significant univariate effects of BMI group on personal growth and purpose in life were computed (see Table 1 for group means). These tests indicated that obese individuals scored significantly lower on both personal growth and purpose in life compared to their normal-weight and overweight counterparts; normal-weight and overweight individuals did not differ significantly on either of these dimensions of psychological well-being.

Table 1. Means on Psychological Well-being Indicators based on Body Weight Groups

	Normal Weight		Overweight		Obese	
	(n = 1335)		(n = 1263)		(n = 724)	
	M	(SD)	M	(SD)	M	(SD)
Positive Relations with Others	16.23	(4.1)	16.15	(4.0)	15.75	(4.2)
Self-Acceptance	16.64	(3.6)	16.60	(3.4)	16.16	(3.5)
Autonomy	16.53	(3.4)	16.46	(3.2)	16.70	(3.3)
Personal Growth**	18.27a	(3.0)	17.82b	(3.1)	17.30ab	(3.4)
Environmental Mastery	16.20	(3.5)	16.17	(3.3)	15.75	(3.5)
Purpose in Life**	16.56a	(3.6)	16.56b	(3.6)	15.93ab	(3.8)

Note: Normal weight=BMI 18.5-24, overweight=BMI 25-29, obese=BMI $\geq$ 30.
Numbers in parentheses are standard deviations.
Higher scores represent higher psychological well-being.
Control variables=age, gender, race, education, marital status, perceived weight.
Main effect for Body Weight Group: multivariate $F[12, 6620]=3.83, p<.001$.
Univariate *F*s significant at $p \leq .01$ (**).
Row means with the same superscripts are significantly different at $p < .05$ or better.

Goal 2: Role of Gender in BMI – Psychological Well-Being Link

Next, we performed a 3 (BMI group: normal-weight, overweight, obese) X 2 (participant's gender) MANCOVA to determine the extent to which the link between BMI and psychological well-being is moderated by gender. In this analysis, we used age, race, education, and marital status as statistical covariates. As can be expected based on the first MANCOVA performed (see first MANCOVA results for Goal 1), we obtained a significant multivariate main effect of BMI group on psychological well-being (F [12, 6616]=3.40, $p <$ .001) with the same pattern of univariate effects. In addition, we obtained a significant multivariate main effect of participants' gender on psychological well-being (F [6, 3307]=17.03, $p < .001$). Univariate effects indicated that, regardless of their BMI group, women scored significantly higher than men on positive relations with others ($F[1,3312]=26.87$, $p < .001$) but scored significantly lower than men on self-acceptance ($F[1,3312]=9.28$, $p < .001$), autonomy ($F[1,3312]=19.64$, $p < .001$), and environmental mastery ($F[1,3312]=23.48$, $p < .001$). More interestingly, however, we found a significant multivariate interaction effect of BMI group X gender on the collective set of psychological well-being indicators ($F[12, 6616]=2.32$, $p < .01$). An examination of the univariate effects indicated significant BMI group X gender interaction effects for three subscales of psychological well-being: positive relations with others ($F[2,3312]=3.77$, $p < .05$), personal growth ($F[2,3312]=6.69$, $p = .001$), and environmental mastery ($F[2,3312]=5.12$, $p < .01$).

Before conducting follow-up analyses for the BMI group X gender interaction effects, we re-ran the above MANCOVA by adding respondents' perceived weight as a statistical covariate to control for the effects of body image in the interactive role of BMI X gender in psychological well-being (see Table 2).

Table 2. Means for Men and Women on Psychological Well-being Indicators based on Body Weight Groups

	Normal Weight		Overweight		Obese	
	Males	Females	Males	Females	Males	Females
	(n=550)	(n=785)	(n=805)	(n=458)	(n=342)	(n=382)
Positive Relations with Othersac	15.59d	16.82dg	15.76e	16.65eh	15.69	15.89gh
Self-Acceptance	16.80	16.53	16.66	16.38	16.55	15.93
AutonomyaPersona l Growthbc	16.78	16.41	16.60	16.17	17.10	16.28
	17.89d	18.39dg	17.92e	17.70eg	17.65f	17.24fg
Environmental MasteryacPurpose in Lifeb	16.28	16.18	16.39	15.73	16.32	15.25
	16.30d	16.55dg	16.63e	16.46eg	16.10	16.15g

The main effects for BMI group (multivariate $F[12,6440]=2.52$, $p < .001$) and gender (multivariate $F[6,3219]=13.52$, $p < .001$) once again achieved statistical significance. The univariate effects for BMI group remained unchanged from those obtained in the second MANCOVA performed for Goal 1 in which the effects of perceived weight were controlled (see Table 1). For the univariate main effects of gender on psychological well-being, once the effects of perceived weight were controlled, the effect for self-acceptance dropped to marginal significance; the remaining three univariate main effects for gender remained significant with women scoring higher than men on positive relations with others ($F[1,3312]=24.37$, $p < .001$) and lower than men on autonomy ($F[1,3312]=16.84$, $p < .001$) and environmental mastery ($F[1,3312]=14.79$, $p < .001$).

The multivariate gender X BMI group interaction effect remained statistically significant in the new analysis ($F[12,6440]=2.30$, $p < .01$). In addition, the three significant univariate interaction effects also persisted: positive relations with others ($F[2,3224]=4.27$, $p < .05$), personal growth ($F[2,3224]=7.67$, $p < .001$), and environmental mastery ($F[2,3224]=5.33$, $p < .01$). We ran two sets of simple effects analyses to determine the source of the significant interaction effect (see Table 2 for a display of the means compared in these simple effects tests). First, we compared men and women on these three psychological well-being indicators in each of the BMI groups using independent samples t-tests (see Figure 1). These tests revealed that 1) on positive relations with others, women scored significantly higher than men in the normal-weight ($t[1333]=4.74$, $p < .001$) and overweight groups ($t[1261]=2.48$, $p < .05$) but no gender differences were found in the obese group; 2) on personal growth, women scored significantly higher than men in the normal-weight group ($t[1333]=2.18$, $p < .001$); however, in the overweight ($t[1261]=-2.48$, $p < .05$) and obese groups ($t[722]=-2.32$, $p < .05$), women scored significantly lower than men and; 3) on environmental mastery, women scored significantly lower than men in the overweight ($t[1261]=-3.86$, $p < .001$) and obese groups ($t[722]=-4.46$, $p < .001$); there were no significant differences in the normal-weight group.

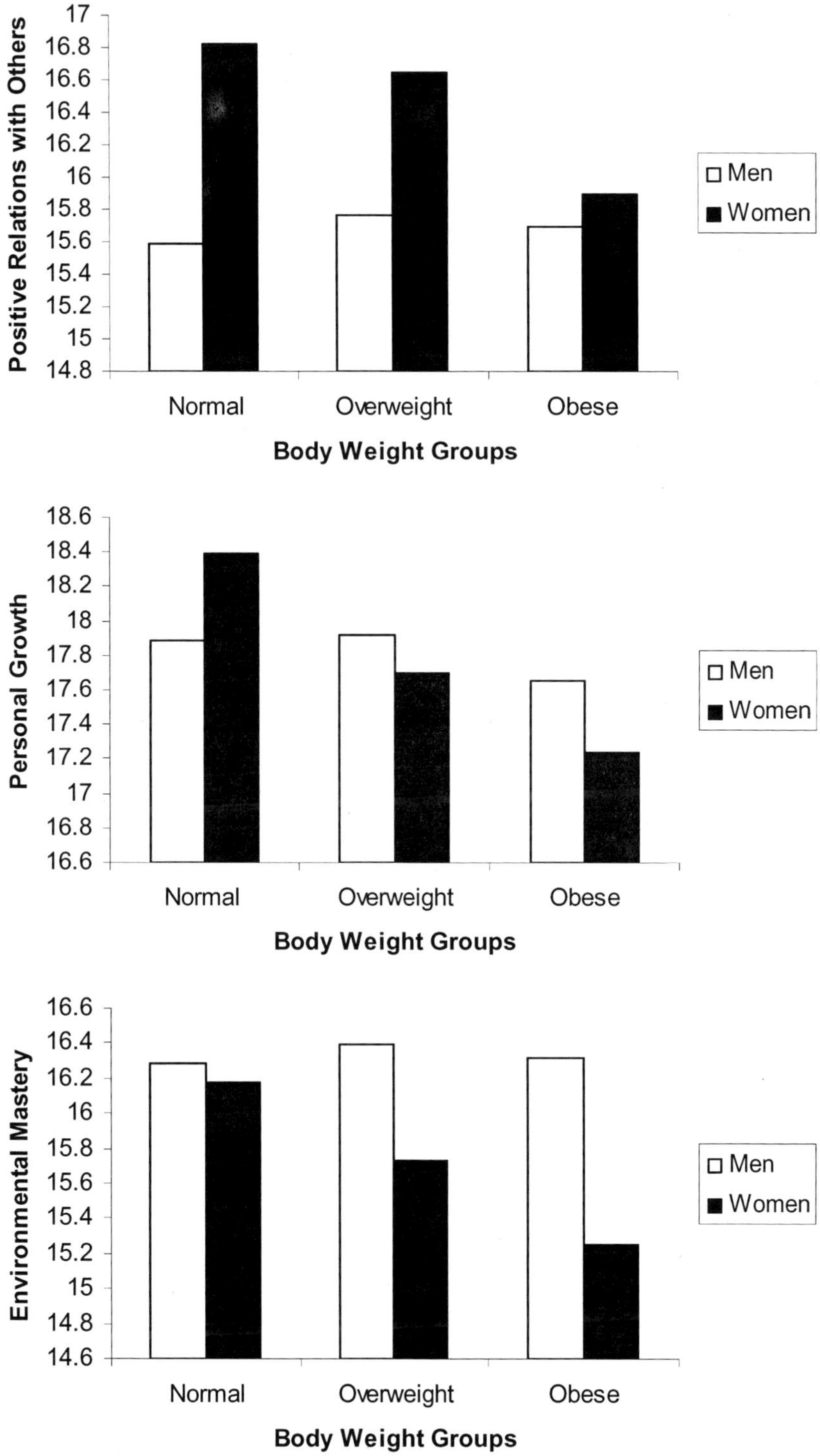

Figure 1. Mean Differences in Psychological Well-being of Men and Women by Body Weight Group.

Second, we compared the three BMI groups separately for men and for women using one-way analysis of variance followed by post-hoc comparisons (see Figure 2).

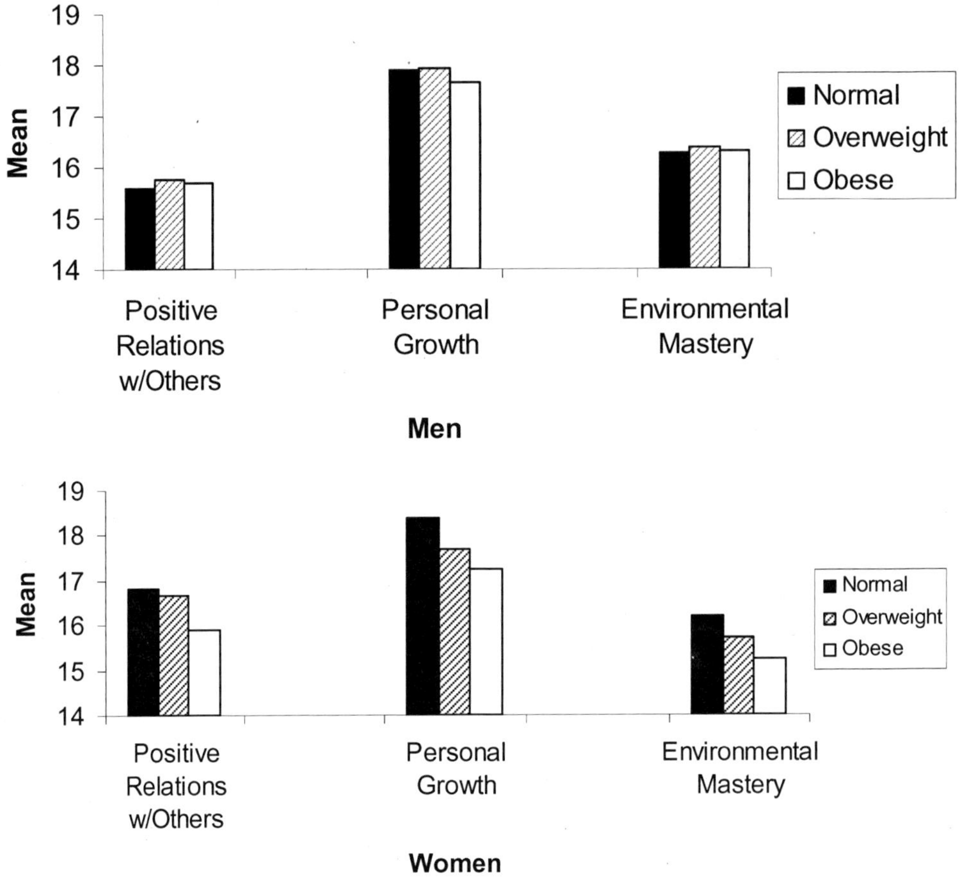

Figure 2. Mean Differences in Psychological Well-being of Normal-Weight, Overweight, and Obese Individuals by Gender.

For men, we found no significant differences based on BMI group (Fs[2,1696]$\leq$2.61, $p >$ .05). For women, however, there were significant differences based on BMI group for each of the three psychological well-being indicators: positive relations with others (F[2,1622]=9.44, $p <$ .001); personal growth (F[2,1622]=26.55, $p <$ .001) and; environmental mastery (F[2,1622]=112.00, $p <$ .001). LSD post-hoc comparisons indicated that obese women scored significantly lower than normal-weight and overweight women on positive relations with others. On personal growth and environmental mastery, all three BMI groups in women were significantly different from one another. Overweight women scored lower on both variables compared with normal-weight women and obese women reported poorer personal growth and environmental mastery than both normal-weight and overweight women.

Discussion

In this study, we examined 1) differences among three groups of adults of varying BMI (normal weight, overweight, and obese individuals) on six dimensions of psychological well-being (Ryff, 1989) and; 2) the extent to which gender moderated the relationship between BMI and psychological well-being in adults. Friedman and Brownell (1995) have emphasized the need for an increase in the number and methodological rigor of studies linking body mass index to psychological well-being. By using a nationally representative probability-based sample of adults that participated in MIDUS (Brim, et al., 2003) and comparing three different BMI groups (including those of normal weight), our study takes an important step in providing new and persuasive evidence that gender differences exist in the psychological well-being of adults who vary on BMI.

First, our results indicate that normal-weight, overweight, and obese adults differ significantly on different dimensions of psychological well-being (Ryff, 1989). After controlling for sociodemographic factors that may play a role in psychological well-being, we found that obese adults scored lower than their normal-weight and/or overweight peers on positive relations with others, personal growth, environmental mastery, and purpose in life; the overall pattern of findings remained the same even after controlling for perceived weight. Our findings substantiate recent findings of poor psychological health among obese adults in studies based on obese treatment-seeking individuals (e.g., Friedman, et al., 2002; Friedman, et al., 2005) and also establish that these levels are lower among obese adults relative to their peers that are of normal-weight or overweight. Our findings also extend those reported by Simon, et al. (2006) linking obesity to a higher lifetime prevalence of mood and anxiety disorders. Our results suggest that higher BMI may have more pervasive and adverse implications for multiple domains of psychological health. While past studies indicate that obese individuals may be more likely to be diagnosed with a psychological disorder at some point in their lives (Heo, et al., 2006; Simon, et al., 2006), it also appears that they may be characterized by lower psychological well-being during adulthood in the form of a poorer sense of purpose in life and a lower capacity for personal growth. To the extent that such poorer psychological well-being, in turn, may place obese individuals at an elevated risk for a mood or anxiety disorder speaks to the clinical significance of our findings.

Second, and perhaps more importantly, our results show that the link between BMI and psychological well-being varies across women and men. We analyzed the interactive effects of gender and BMI on psychological well-being in two ways. First, when we compared women and men on psychological well-being within each BMI category, we found that normal-weight women had similar levels of (on environmental mastery) or better (on positive relations with others and personal growth) psychological well-being compared to their normal-weight male counterparts. In contrast, being overweight or obese appears to be linked to significantly worse psychological well-being for women relative to men in the same BMI categories. Our analyses revealed that obese women do not have the advantage enjoyed by their normal-weight peers over their male counterparts on positive relations with others and they score significantly lower on both environmental mastery and personal growth than obese men. The findings for overweight women represent fewer clear-cut disadvantages for psychological well-being – whereas overweight women have lower environmental mastery than their male overweight peers, they are not significantly different on personal growth and have more positive relations with others than do overweight men. Next, we compared the different BMI groups separately for women and men. We found a clear linear and stepwise pattern of worse psychological well-being by BMI group for women such that obese women had lower positive relations with others, environmental mastery, and personal growth than overweight women who, in turn, had lower environmental mastery and personal growth than normal-weight women. These findings support past research that has found greater anxiety reported by women than by men about becoming overweight (Cash and Brown, 1989; Muth and Cash, 1997). Our results are particularly important because we controlled for perceptions of body weight (i.e., viewing oneself to be very underweight, of the right weight, or very overweight), indicating that gender differences in the link between BMI and psychological well-being are not simply explained by differences in body image, a construct on which women typically score less favorably than do men (e.g., Franzoi and Koehler, 1998; McKinley, 1999).

One explanation for our finding that being of normal-weight is associated with psychological benefits and that being obese is associated with psychological risks for women over men comes in the form of prevailing gender-differentiated cultural norms surrounding body weight. For Westernized cultures in particular, femininity – specifically thinness – is closely related to physical attractiveness. Research has found that being of slender weight is the most salient correlate of positive appearance evaluation in women and that lower BMI is associated with greater rated physical attractiveness among women (Cash and Henry, 1995). In comparison, for men greater BMI is linked to greater power and strength inasmuch as the ideal masculine body type is a muscular one (Grogan, and Richards, 2002). Research has indicated that women are likely to internalize cultural norms linking thinness to physical attractiveness and thus, view themselves more critically then do men (McKinley and Hyde, 1996). Rodin, Silberstein, and Striegel-Moore (1985), for example, observed that body weight dissatisfaction amongst women in Westernized cultures has become a "normative discontent." Such cultural norms are readily transmitted through sociocultural discourse via the mass media. For example, in a content analysis of several primetime television situation comedies, Fouts and Burggraf (2000) found that male characters directed significantly more negative comments about or to heavier female characters compared with below-average weight female characters and that such comments were systematically linked with eliciting audience laughter.

Another possible explanation for our obtained gender differences may emerge from stigma theory applications to overweight and obese individuals (e.g., Allon, 1981; Faulkner, et al., 1999; Friedman, et al., 2005; Puhl and Brownell, 2001; Sarlio-Lahteenkorva, Stunkard, and Rissanen, 1995). It is possible, for example, that the nature and intensity of the stigma experienced by obese individuals varies by gender and that women experience stronger social stigma for being overweight relative to their male counterparts. Indirect support for this emerges from Neumark-Sztainer, et al.'s (2002) study that examined the experience of teasing in a population of adolescents. They found that overweight girls in particular reported that they were especially bothered by others' teasing. Likewise, in a series of focus groups, Cossrow, Jeffery, and McGuire (2001), found that women participants reported a greater number and variety of negative experiences related to their excess weight compared to men.

These experiences encompassed teasing, slurs and insults, harassment, negative judgments and assumptions, and perceived discrimination related to their weight. In another study, Chen and Brown (2005) found that, relative to obese men, obese women are more likely to experience stigmatization by men during a sexual partner choice task. We recommend that future research focus on exploring differences in stigmatizing social interactions and experiences of overweight and obese women vs. men as a potential explanation for gender differences in overweight and obese individuals' psychological well-being.

Conclusion

Our study indicates that gender clearly moderates the relationship between BMI and psychological well-being. It is important to point out, however, that our study is based on cross-sectional data and, thus, we cannot draw conclusions about the direction of causal relationships linking BMI and psychological well-being. Nevertheless, regardless of whether excessive body weight leads to poorer psychological well-being or the reverse, our results confirm that women and men vary in the strength of the association between these variables with the association being stronger for women than for men. Another limitation of our study is that in MIDUS (Brim, et al., 2003) BMI was calculated based on self-reports of weight and height obtained from the participants rather than on objective evaluations. It is possible, therefore, that MIDUS respondents did not accurately report their vital statistics. However, at least in the case of self-reports of weight, heavier individuals may be likely to underreport rather than over-report their weight. For example, a study by Koslowski, Scheinberg, Bleich, and Mark,(1994) found that participants who weighed more tended to underreport their weight. In light of this tendency for heavier individuals to underreport their weight, it is likely that we would find even stronger moderating effects of gender in the relationship between BMI and psychological well-being. Nevertheless, we urge future studies to use objective assessments of vital statistics when measuring body weight.

In closing, we would like to highlight that our study is marked by several strengths that enhance our confidence in its findings. We used data from a large, nationally-representative probability-based, non-clinical sample of adults, we examined the moderating role of gender in the association between BMI and psychological well-being after controlling for sociodemographic variables, and we used perceived weight as a statistical covariate. In doing so, we make original contributions to the intersecting literatures on body weight, body image, and gender differences in health.

References

Allon, N. (1981). The stigma of overweight in everyday life. In B. Wolman (Ed.), *Psychological aspects of obesity: A handbook* (pp. 130-174). New York: Van Nostrand Rheinhold.

Brim, O. G., Baltes, P. B., Bumpass, L. L., Cleary, P. D., Featherman, D. L., Hazzard, W. R., et al. (2003). National Survey of Midlife Development in the United States (MIDUS),

1995-1996 [Computer File]. Second ICPSR version. Ann Arbor, MI: DataStat Inc./Boston, MA: Harvard Medical School, Department of Health Care Policy [producers], 1996. Ann Arbor, MI: Inter-University Consortium for Political and Social Research [distributor], 2003.

Carr, D. and Friedman, M. A. (2006). Body weight and the quality of interpersonal relationships. *Social Psychology Quarterly, 69,* 127-149.

Cash, T. F., and Brown, T. A. (1989). Gender and body image: Stereotypes and realities. *Sex Roles, 21,* 361-373. Cash, T. F. and Henry, P. E (1995). Women's body images: The result of a national survey in the U.S.A. *Sex Roles, 33,* 19-28.

Chen E. Y., and Brown, M. (2005). Obesity stigma in sexual relationships. *Obesity Research, 13,* 1393-1397.

Cossrow, N. H. F., Jeffery, R. W., and McGuire, M. W. (2001). Understanding weight stigmatization: A focus group study. *Journal of Nutrition Education, 33,* 208-214.

Davison, T. E., and McCabe, M. P. (2005). Relationships between men's and women's body image and their psychological, social, and sexual functioning. *Sex Roles, 52,* 463 (13).

Faulkner, N. H., French, S. A., Jeffery, R. W., Neumark-Sztainer, D., Sherwood, N. E., and Morton, N. (1999). Mistreatment due to weight: Prevalence and sources of perceived mistreatment in women and men. *Obesity Research, 7,* 572-576.

Flegal, K. M., Carroll, M. D., Ogden, C. L., and Johnson, C. L. (2002). Prevalence and trends in obesity among US adults, 1999-2000. *Journal of the American Medical Association, 288,* 1723-1727.

Fouts, G., and Burggraf, K. (2000). Television situation comedies: Female weight, male negative comments, and audience reactions. *Sex Roles, 42,* 925-932.

Franzoi, S.L., and Herzog, M.E. (1986). The Body Esteem Scale: A convergent and discriminant validity study. *Journal of Personality Assessment, 50,* 24-31.

Franzoi, S. L., and Koehler, V. (1998). Age and gender differences in body attitudes: A comparison of young and elderly adults. *International Journal of Aging and Human Development, 47,* 1-10.

Friedman, K. E., Reichmann, S. K., Constanzo, P. R., and Musante, G. J. (2002). Body image partially mediates the relationship between obesity and psychological distress. *Obesity Research, 10,* 33-41.

Friedman, K. E., Reichmann, S. K., Costanzo, P. R., Zelli, A., Ashmore, J. A., and Musante, J. G. (2005). Weight stigmatization and ideological beliefs: Relation to psychological functioning in obese adults. *Obesity Research, 13,* 907-916.

Friedman, M. A., and Brownell, K. D. (1995). Psychological correlates of obesity: Moving to the next research generation. *Psychological Bulletin, 177,* 3-20.

Grogan, S., and Richards, H. (2002). Body image: Focus groups with boys and men. *Men and Masculinities, 4,* 219-232.

Heo, M., Pietrobelli, A., Fontaine, K. R., Sirey, J.A., and Faith, M. S. (2006). Depressive mood and obesity in US adults: Comparison and moderation by age, sex, and race. *International Journal of Obesity, 30,* 513-519.

Koslowski, M., Scheinberg, Z., Bleich, A., and Mark, M. (1994). Predicting actual weight from self-report data. *Educational and Psychological Measurement, 54,* 168-173.

Linde, J. A., Jefferey, R. W., Levy, R. L., Sherwood, N. E., Utter, J., Pronk, N. P., et al. (2004). Binge eating disorder, weight control self-efficacy, and depression in overweight men and women. *International Journal of Overweight and Obesity, 28*, 418-425.

McKinley, N. M. (1999). Women and objectified body consciousness: Mothers' and daughters' body experience in cultural, developmental, and familial context. *Developmental Psychology, 33*, 760-769.

McKinley, N. M., and Hyde, J. S. (1996). The objectified body consciousness scale: Development and validation. *Psychology of Women Quarterly, 20*, 181-215.

Muth, J. L., and Cash, T. F. (1997). Body-image attitudes: What difference does gender make? *Journal of Applied Social Psychology, 27*, 1438-1452.

National Heart, Lung, and Blood Institute (1998). *Clinical guidelines on the identification, evaluation, and treatment of overweight and obesity in adults: The evidence report (Publication 98-4803).* National Institutes of Health: Bethesda, MD.

Neumark-Sztainer, D., Falkner, N., Story, M., Perry, C., Hannan, P.J., and Mulert, S. (2002). Weight-teasing among adolescents: Correlations with weight status and disordered eating behaviors. *International Journal of Obesity, 26*, 123-131.

Nunnally, J. M. (1978). *Psychometric theory*. New York: McGraw-Hill.

Ogden, C. L., Carroll, M. D., Curtin, L. R., McDowell, M. A., Tabak, C. J., et al. (2006). Prevalence of overweight and obesity in the United States, 1999-2004. *Journal of the American Medical Association, 295*, 1549-1555.

O'Neil, P. M., and Jarrell, M. P. (1992). Psychological aspects of obesity and dieting. In T. A. Wadden and T. B. Van Itallie (Eds.), *Treatment of the seriously obese patient* (pp. 252- 270). New York: Guilford Press.

Puhl, R., and Brownell, K. D. (2001). Bias, discrimination, and obesity. *Obesity Research, 9*, 788-805.

Rodin, J., Silberstein, L. R., and Striegel-Moore, R. H. (1985). Women and weight: A normative discontent. *Nebraska Symposium on Motivation, 32,* 267-307.

Ryff, C. D. (1989). Happiness is everything, or is it? Explorations on the meaning of psychological well-being. *Journal of Personality and Social Psychology, 57*, 1069-1081.

Ryff, C. D., and Keyes, C. M. (1995). The structure of psychological well-being revisited. *Journal of Personality and Social Psychology, 69,* 719-727.

Sarlio-Lahteenkorva, S., Stunkard, A., and Rissanen, A. (1995). Psychosocial factors and quality of life in obesity. *International Journal of Obesity, 6*, S1-5.

Simon, G.E., Von Korff, M., Saunders, K., Miglioretti, D.L., Crane, P.K., Van Belle, G., et al. (2006). Association between obesity and psychiatric disorders in the US adult population. *Archives of General Psychiatry, 63,* 824-830.

Stunkard, A.J., Faith, M.S., and Allison, K.C. (2003). Depression and obesity. *Biological*

Wadden, T. A., and Stunkard, A. J. (1993). Psychosocial consequences of obesity and dieting- research and clinical findings. In A. J. Stunkard and T. A. Wadden (Eds.), *Obesity theory and therapy* (pp. 163-177). New York: Raven Press.

Weaver, A. D., and Byers, E. S. (2006). The relationships among body image, body mass index, exercise, and sexual functioning in heterosexual women. *Psychology of Women Quarterly, 30,* 333-339.

World Health Organization (2002). *The World Health Report 2002: Reducing risks, promoting healthy life*. Geneva, Switzerland: World Health Organization.

In: New Directions in Aging Research
Editor: Ruby R. Brougham, pp. 39-56
ISBN 978-1-60741-976-1
© 2009 Nova Science Publishers, Inc.

Chapter 3

Dyadic Interventions for Persons with Early-Stage Dementia: A Cognitive Rehabilitative Focus

Maureen Schmitter-Edgecombe, Shital Pavawalla, Joni T. Howard, Lisa Howell and Alicia Rueda*
Washington State University, Pullman, Washington, USA

Abstract

Non-drug therapies are increasingly being recommended in conjunction with drug therapies in the treatment of Alzheimer's disease (AD). Recent advances in accurately diagnosing the early symptoms of dementia have led to the suggestion that interventions that include both members of the care dyad may represent an optimal approach. In this chapter, we first review the literature with regards to dyadic interventions that have been used with AD and early-stage dementia patients. We then report on pilot work conducted in our laboratory which blends cognitive rehabilitation with a dyadic intervention aimed at strengthening the relationship between the individual with early-stage dementia and their caregiver. This blended dyadic cognitive rehabilitation approach has the potential to meet the challenge of helping early-stage dementia patients and their caregivers maintain hope, while also facilitating adjustment and adaptation to the changes that dementia brings.

Introduction

Up to 4.5 million people in the U.S. currently suffer from Alzheimer's disease (AD), with the number of new cases each year expected to double between 1995 and 2050 (from 377,000

* Correspondence concerning this article should be addressed to Maureen Schmitter-Edgecombe, Department of Psychology, Washington State University, Pullman, Washington 99164-4820. Phone: 509-335-0170. FAX: 509-335-5043. Electronic mail may be sent to schmitter-e@wsu.edu

to 959,000) if no preventative treatments become available (Hebert, Scherr, Bienias, Bennett, and Evans, 2003). The costs associated with AD put a heavy economic and emotional burden on society. The Lewin Group (2004) estimated that total Medicare spending on AD patients will increase from $62 billion in 2000 to more than $1 trillion by 2050. Significant economic, emotional, psychological, and physical costs are also associated with caring for patients with AD, with a rapidly increasing number of AD family caregivers being at increased risk for health problems (Vitaliano, Echeverria, Shelkey, Zhang, and Scanlan, 2007). Of considerable importance are interventions that can delay the disability associated with AD, decrease caregiver burden, and reduce the health care costs associated with treatment of both AD patients and their caregivers.

Increasingly, a combination of drug and non-drug interventions is being advocated to optimize everyday functioning in persons with AD (De Vreese, Neri, Fioravanti, Belloi, and Zanetti, 2001; Requena, et al., 2004). However, the efficacy of non-drug interventions has been repeatedly questioned since early attempts at cognitive rehabilitation for AD patients in the late 1960s (e.g., APA, 1997; Rabins, 1996). As a striking example, after reviewing the cognitive intervention literature up to the early 1990s, the steering committee of the American Psychiatric Association (APA, 1997) concluded that "cognition-oriented treatments are not supported by efficacy data and also have the potential to produce adverse effects". Currently, the majority of non-drug interventions for AD involve either treating only the AD patients or providing caregiver support and education separately from the patients. With recent advances in accurately diagnosing the early symptoms of dementia, interventions that include both members of the care dyad may represent a more optimal approach (Whitlatch, Judge, Zarit, and Femia, 2006). Such an approach offers the potential to attend to the needs of both partners and to maintain the dyadic relationship through dealing more effectively with adjustments presented by memory and behavioral deficits associated with AD. In addition, most individuals with early-stage dementia want to be proactive, demonstrate the ability for new learning and can utilize intact cognitive skills to aid in compensating for impaired abilities. These points underscore a clear need for evidence-based cognitive rehabilitation in the treatment of early-stage dementia (Clare and Woods, 2004).

We begin this chapter with a brief discussion of caregiver-centered treatments and patient-centered interventions for AD. Consistent with the recent work of others (e.g., Whitlatch, et al., 2006; Logsdon, McCurry, and Teri, 2007), we suggest that interventions aimed at working with both members of the dyad may be a more optimal approach to treatment for individuals with early-stage dementia. Next, we review the literature with regards to dyadic interventions that have been used with AD and early-stage dementia patients. We then report on pilot work conducted in our laboratory which blends cognitive rehabilitation with a dyadic intervention aimed at strengthening the relationship between the individual with early-stage dementia and the caregiver. This blended dyadic cognitive rehabilitation approach has the potential to meet the challenge of helping early-stage dementia patients and their caregivers maintain hope, while also facilitating adjustment and adaptation to the changes that dementia brings. In the final section, we discuss strengths and challenges to this type of intervention and make practical suggestions for future treatment implementation.

Cognitive-centered and Patient-centered Interventions

While it is well-known that AD has a profound impact on both the patient's life and the caregiver's life (Zarit and Leitsch, 2001), as stated earlier, interventions have generally targeted either the patient or the caregiver individually (Onor, et al., 2007; Whitlatch, et al., 2006). Studies evaluating caregiver-centered treatments have reported a variety of effective interventions, reflecting varied theoretical orientations (e.g., cognitive-behavioral, brief psychodynamic; Marriott, Donaldson, Tarrier, and Burns, 2000; Teri, Logsdon, Uomoto, and McCurry, 1997) and different procedural formats (e.g., support groups and psychoeducational groups; Coon, Thompson, Steffen, Sorocco, and Gallgher-Thompson, 2003). The primary goal and associated outcome measures for many of these studies have focused on whether the intervention can successfully help the caregiver reduce their depression and anger (Akkerman and Ostwald, 2004; Steffen and Berger, 2000). In contrast, patient-centered interventions have included pharmacological treatment and rehabilitation with a range of techniques, including reminiscence therapy, cognitive stimulation techniques, and occupational therapy (Baines, Saxby, and Ehlert, 1987; Requena, et al., 2004). The primary outcome for these patient-focused studies has been to evaluate whether the interventions can improve or maintain the patient's cognitive status and residual functional abilities (Cahn-Weiner, Malloy, Rebok, and Ott, 2003; Loewenstein, Acevedo, Czaja, and Duara, 2004), with measures of caregiver outcomes relatively ignored (Brodaty, 2007). For those studies that have directed treatment towards both members of the care dyad (Smits, et al., 2007), patients and caregivers typically received different interventions (e.g., Berger, et al., 2004; Onor ,et al., 2007). This approach of treating the caregiver and care recipient separately is understandable in that it reflects an awareness of the differing cognitive status and needs of the AD patients and their caregivers. However, given the intact awareness and higher cognitive skill levels of most early-stage dementia patients, it raises the possibility that interventions aimed at treating both members of the care dyad may represent a more optimal approach to treatment for early-stage dementia (Whitlatch, et al., 2006).

Dyadic Interventions

In an early series of studies, Quayhagen and colleagues (e.g., Quayhagen, Quayhagen, Corbeil, Roth, and Rogers, 1995; Quayhagen and Quayhagen, 2001) investigated the efficacy of a cognitive stimulation program for persons with a confirmed diagnosis of possible or probable AD. The cognitive stimulation program was implemented in the home by the caregiver. Caregivers and care recipients were trained together in weekly in-home sessions with members of the intervention team. The intervention consisted of 60 minutes of daily active cognitive stimulation centered on memory, problem-solving, and conversational activities. In this initial study (Quayhagen, et al. 1995), outcome measures were directed solely towards the AD patient with the results supporting the viability of cognitive rehabilitation interventions with dementia patients. More specifically, Quayhagen and colleagues (1995) found that, in contrast to a wait-list control group that showed decline and a placebo group (passive activities) that remained static, care recipients in the active cognitive stimulation group improved in cognitive and behavioral performance with treatment. In later studies, Quayhagen and colleagues (2001) extended outcome measurement to the caregivers and documented beneficial effects of the home-based stimulation program for caregivers. Most notably, caregivers endorsed being more satisfied with their interactions with the care recipient, and identified enhanced communication and interaction as a major benefit of the home-based cognitive stimulation intervention (Corbeil, Quayhagen and Quayhagen, 1999; Quayhagen and Quayhagen, 2001). Throughout the intervention, the caregiver was assisted with interacting more effectively with the patient through observation of the interactions modeled by the research/training team during the weekly sessions.

In another study, Quayhagen and colleagues (Quayhagen, et al., 2000) evaluated four non-pharmacological interventions for the treatment of dementia: cognitive stimulation, dyadic counseling, dual supportive seminar, and early-stage day care. The care recipients were evaluated at baseline and post-intervention (3 months) on cognitive status while the caregivers were assessed on marital interaction, emotional status, and physical health, as well as stress, coping, and social support. Quantitative data analyses revealed that caregivers in the cognitive stimulation group reported a decrease in depressive symptoms and that patients demonstrated improvement over time in cognitive outcomes. No other intervention led to positive changes in the cognitive status of the patient. However, caregivers in the early-stage day care and dual supportive seminar groups reported a significant decrease in hostility and use of negative coping strategies, respectively. Analysis of the qualitative evaluation data revealed that enhancing communication was a major benefit identified by caregivers in the dyadic counseling group and by caregivers in the cognitive stimulation group, who also identified mental stimulation as a major benefit. Consistent with the differential focal points of treatment, caregivers in the early-stage dementia day group identified enhanced emotional involvement as a major benefit. In addition, while caregivers in the dual-supportive seminar group identified acquiring insight and building caregiver relationships as major benefits, they also reported decreased patient morale possibly due to the discussion of dementia symptoms and progression that occurred in the group (Quayhagen, et al., 2000). These findings suggest that additional benefits can be gained from working with the care dyad in a way that not only facilitates adjustment and adaptation to the changes that dementia brings, but that also aids in maintaining hope and promoting functional independence for dementia patients through cognitive rehabilitation.

A handful of more recent studies have approached dementia intervention with the specific aim of strengthening the care dyad but without a rehabilitation focus. Based on anecdotal and qualitative data, Zarit and colleagues (Zarit, Femia, Watson, Rice-Oeschger, and Kakos, 2004) reported that a 10-session group program (Memory Club) designed to empower both members of the care dyad to participate jointly in managing current problems and planning for the future appeared to be a promising program. One of the most helpful aspects of the Memory club described by both members of the care dyad was the opportunity to learn from and share feelings and experiences with other people in similar situations. This same group of researchers also recently completed a feasibility study of a structured, 9-session protocol for one-on-one and dyadic counseling for care recipients in the early-stage of dementia and their caregivers (Whitlatch, et al., 2006). All sessions were held in the participants' home and were led by trained counselors. The program was designed to strengthen the relationship bond and engage both members of the care dyad in a dialogue about future preferences for care, thereby addressing some of the worry and uncertainty experienced by each member of the care dyad. Feasibility and acceptability data indicated that dyads enrolled in the program successfully completed the full intervention and were highly satisfied.

Preliminary data was also recently reported for two, ongoing randomized controlled clinical trials investigating the value of couples counseling (Epstein, Auclair, and Mittelman, 2007) and the efficacy of a time-limited support group (Logsdon, et al., 2007) for persons in the early-stages of dementia and their caregivers. Both clinical trials shared a common goal of improving quality of life for individuals with dementia and their families. Preliminary data from both studies appears positive, with the time-limited support group intervention leading to improved quality of life and decreased family conflict following support group participation (Logsdon, et al., 2007). These studies, though preliminary, are suggestive in showing that psychoeducational and support treatment for care dyads may confer benefits both for individual members of the dyad as well as the overall relationship.

Dyadic Cognitive Rehabilitative Intervention

The combined findings from the work discussed above suggest that significant benefits could be gained by linking cognitive rehabilitation strategies with a dyadic intervention aimed at strengthening the dyad relationship. Such benefits would include not only improving the relationship of the care dyad and the mental health and quality of life for each member, but also increasing the cognitive and functional abilities of the care recipient. This type of intervention would also meet an identified challenge for working with early-stage dementia patients, specifically, helping these individuals find ways of maintaining hope and strengthening their sense of self while also facilitating adjustment and adaptation to the changes that dementia brings (Clare, 2002). The cognitive rehabilitation component of the intervention would provide members of the care dyad with something positive to focus on and may reduce expressed feelings of helplessness and frustration qualitatively reported in some early-stage dementia support group programs (Goldsilver and Gruneir, 2001; Quayhagen, et al., 2000). In recent pilot work we examined the efficacy of a dyadic cognitive rehabilitative intervention which focused on teaching persons with early-stage dementia and their caregiver how to use a memory notebook.

We focused the rehabilitation component on memory impairment for several reasons. First, individuals with early-stage dementia and their caregivers often report frustration associated with the memory problems that the care recipient is experiencing and request assistance. Memory impairment is one of the earliest and most problematic symptoms of AD. Memory difficulties can lower a patient's self-confidence and lead to withdrawal from activities (Ballard, Bannister, and Oyebode, 1996; Ballard, Boyle, Bowler, and Lindesay, 1996). Caregivers are also affected by the patient's memory problems in everyday life and by the strain and frustration experienced by the patient (Zarit and Edwards, 1996). It has been advocated that providing help with memory problems is critical to the management of AD

(Maeda, 2005). Supporting this sentiment, a recent study found that for persons with early-stage dementia the greatest magnitude of change in everyday functioning was associated with functional abilities that relied on memory (e.g., remembering current date, remembering appointments; Farias, et al., 2006).

Second, within the cognitive rehabilitation literature, several approaches to treating memory impairment have been identified as effective with AD. For example, vanishing cues, procedural memory activation, the spaced-retrieval technique, and errorless learning have all been used successfully with AD patients to teach domain-specific old or new knowledge (Camp, Foss, O'Hanlon and Stevens, 1996; Camp, et al., 1996; Clare, Wilson, Breen, and Hodges, 1999) and to intervene with everyday memory problems (Clare, et al., 2000; Farina, et al., 2002). These techniques have been suggested to be successful because they engage processes that lie outside of the declarative memory system and are related to spared memory functions (e.g., implicit memory; De Vreese ,et al., 2001; Acevedo and Loewenstein, 2007). The significance of engaging processes related to spared memory functions is indirectly supported by a recent subgroup analysis of memory-impaired participants from the Advanced Training for Independent and Vital Elderly (ACTIVE) trial. This analysis showed that, unlike persons without memory impairment, persons with memory impairment failed to benefit from the memory training intervention, which focused on learning strategies that required explicit, conscious, associative linking (i.e., declarative memory; Unverzagt, et al., 2007). External memory aids have also proven valuable for helping AD patients to compensate for everyday difficulties that result from memory loss. For example, memory books and other assistive devices such as timers have been found to be effective in decreasing repetitive questions (Bourgeois, et al., 2003), reducing behavioral excesses (Holmes, 2000), and in supporting daily functioning in persons with AD (Langill and Schmitter-Edgecombe, 2007; Quittre, Oliver, and Salmon, 2005).

We modeled our approach to teaching the care dyad to use a memory notebook after a systematic learning method that was introduced by Sohlberg and Mateer (1989) and used by our laboratory in a previous study with traumatic brain-injured patients (Schmitter-Edgecombe, Fahy, Whelan, and Long, 1995). In our initial work with a single-dyad (Langill and Schmitter-Edgecombe, 2007), we found that a 71-year old female (EC) with very mild dementia was able to successfully learn to automatize journaling in, and referring to, a memory notebook. EC, a former elementary school teacher, was diagnosed with very mild dementia approximately three years prior to participating in memory notebook training with her spousal caregiver. At the time of the intervention, she was experiencing significant problems in the areas of new learning and memory (Borderline to Impaired range performances), while the remainder of her cognitive skills remained relatively intact (generally Average range or above). EC was also aware of her memory difficulties and was highly motivated to develop and implement new strategies in her everyday life to help her compensate for memory loss.

The primary goal of the memory notebook training was to provide EC and her husband with a way to help EC compensate for impairments in her declining memory system, and enable her to continue to participate independently in her daily activities in a meaningful manner. Over the course of 17 sessions, EC was first taught a structured, organized means to record her daily events; this was designed to aid her retrospective memory by enabling her to refer back to recently completed activities. She was then taught to use the notebook to schedule, plan, and carry out future activities, thus aiding her prospective memory, or ability to remember to complete future actions. We have observed that the act of writing in the memory notebook is itself an important cognitive activity which helps to focus the individual's attention on the information to be recorded and aids in increasing repetition of information in a multi-modal format. The periodic review of significant events recorded in the memory notebook may also help to strengthen memories through processes similar to those seen with spaced-retrieval techniques or more recently reported with use of SenseCam technology (Berry, et al., 2007).

To examine the impact of the memory notebook treatment, we assessed for depression, symptom distress, and everyday memory lapses at pre-treatment and post-treatment, as well as at 2-, 6-, and 12-month follow-ups. On a measure of global distress (i.e., Symptom Checklist 90-Revised; Derogatis, 1975), EC demonstrated a 50% reduction in symptom endorsement from pre-treatment to post-treatment, and this gain was maintained at the 12-month follow-up. No notable changes were seen in symptom endorsement on a measure of depression (i.e., Geriatric Depression Scale; Yesavage, et al., 1983), however, ECs scores fell within normal limits on this measure at all time points. Pre-treatment (mild depression) to post-treatment (normal range) changes in endorsement of depressive symptoms were observed for EC's husband. In comparison to pre-treatment, a decrease in everyday memory lapses (documented by a 7-day daily checklist of memory lapses completed by EC and her husband) was also seen at post-treatment and maintained at 2- and 6-month follow-ups, over which period EC engaged in notebook use on 80% of the days. At the 12-month follow-up, a drop in memory notebook entries was found suggesting that booster sessions may be needed every few month. As assessed by a brief neuropsychological battery, EC's overall cognitive status remained relatively stable over the course of the year.

The success of this memory notebook system in helping EC and her husband better manage the cognitive, emotional, and functional changes associated with early-stage dementia led us to initiate a multi-dyad group (Schmitter-Edgecombe, Howard, Pavawalla, Howell, and Rueda, submitted). The group contained five individuals with very mild dementia (4 females, 1 male) and four spousal caregivers who served as coaches (1 female, 3 males). The group participated in 14 treatment sessions administered 2x per week over 7 weeks. All early-stage dementia participants (a) scored a 0.5 on the Clinical Dementia Rating scale (CDR; Hughes, Berg, Danzinger, Coben, and Martin, 1982; Morris, 1993; Morris, et al., 1991), consistent with a very mild dementia; (b) reported memory impairment of 6 months or longer, which was corroborated by performance on memory measures falling 1.5 SD below the mean of age and education matched peers; (c) scored above 24 on the Mini Mental Status Examination (MMSE; Folstein, Folstein, and McHugh, 1975) and, with the exception of memory, demonstrated relatively preserved functions in other cognitive domains assessed through the neuropsychological screening (i.e., attention, language, executive abilities); (d) showed awareness for their memory difficulties, and (e) expressed a desire for treatment.

The purpose of each of the five memory notebook sections introduced during the course of the intervention is described in Table 1. Figure 1 also provides a graphic of the daily log section of the memory notebook.

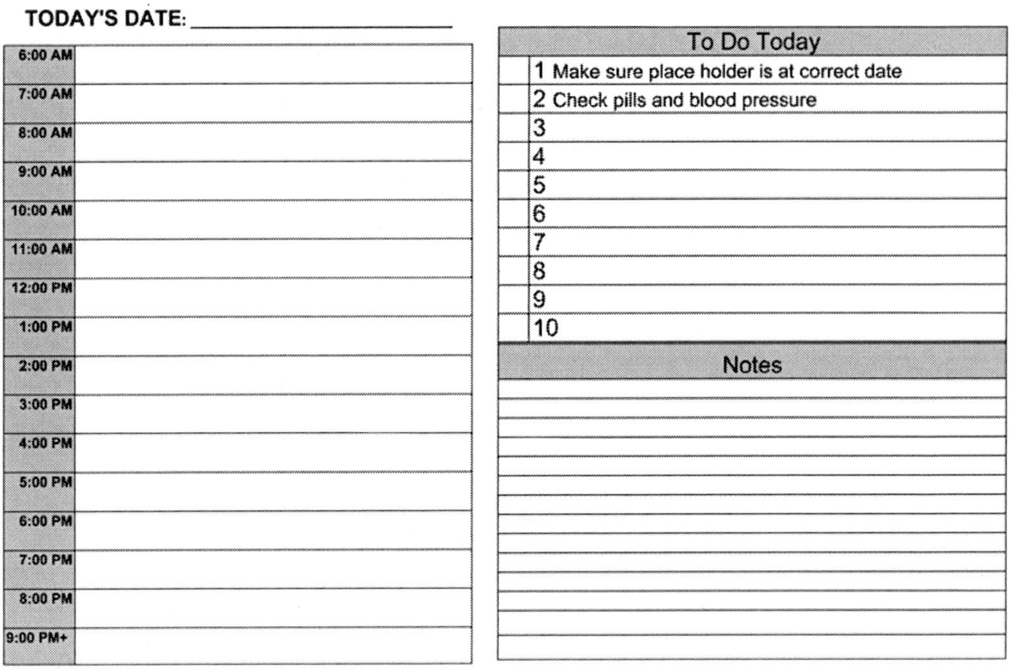

Figure 1. Example Daily Log pages. Activities needing completion each day can be customized and pre-printed in the To Do Today section or Hourly Daily Log.

Table 1. Notebook Sections and Purpose

Notebook Sections	Purpose
Daily Log	Used to record, store, and retrieve information about daily activities. Contains forms for charting hourly information and scheduling activities/appointments. Contains forms for prioritizing a to-do-today list.
Calendar	Used for recording appointments and retrieving information about important meetings and upcoming events.
Personal Notes	Used for recording important personal information such as medications, addresses, birthdays etc.
Current Work	Used for recording specific procedures about work assignments that may be needed at a later date.
Personal Goals	Used to record, store, and retrieve information relevant to the personal goals of the individual (e.g., creating an autobiography).

Treatment involved modeling, psycho-education, and the completion of activities directed by therapists that were incorporated into nine learning activities packets. The learning activities packets included a set of goals and in-session activities, as well as homework assignments that assisted the dyads and singleton in learning to use and incorporate the memory notebook into their everyday lives. Teaching of the memory notebook proceeded in four stages: anticipation, acquisition, application, and adaptation. The title and primary goals of the learning activities packets introduced in each stage are shown in Table 2. The notebooks were regularly reviewed by the four therapists to evaluate and encourage skill development. Although the group format was paramount, each care dyad and the singleton were assigned a therapist, so as to increase personal attention to specific needs and place greater accountability upon participants to carry out assigned homework tasks. Modifications to the notebooks for personal needs were routinely discussed. Participants were also provided with an alarm to cue them to regularly use the notebook.

Table 2. Learning Activities Packets and their Purpose

Learning Activities Packet	Primary Purpose/Goal
ANTICIPATION	
Memory	Provide psychoeducation about memory; increase understanding of how changes in the brain affect behavior; identify compensatory and coping strategies in use by dyads; pique interest in memory strategy.
ACQUISITION	
Your Memory Notebook	Provide psychoeducation about internal and external memory strategies; help dyads identify and problem solve ways to minimize common stumbling blocks to memory notebook use (e.g., embarrassment, forget to use it).
Recording Information in your Notebook	Teach use of daily log; demonstrate how referring to daily log can aid everyday retrospective memory difficulties; teach strategies for writing meaningful and detailed notebook entries; help identify strategies (e.g., activity completion) or aids (e.g., alarm) that will support frequent notebook use.
Using Your Daily Log	Teach use of the to-do-today section of the daily log for creating a list of tasks to complete; discuss how scheduling an appointment with one's self can aid completion of everyday activities.
APPLICATION	
Quality of Life	Discuss concept of quality of life; help identify and schedule in notebook activities to enhance quality of life; reinforce use of the to-do-today section of the daily log for aiding in implementation of improved quality of life activities.
Documenting and Transferring	Teach system for documenting activity completion and transferring incomplete activities to the next day; help dyads integrate notebook use with other strategies in use.
Scheduling Appointments	Practice identifying and recording needed information for new appointments (e.g. time, date, directions, things need to bring, etc.); discuss how notebook can aid with prospective memory difficulties.
ADAPTATION	
Personal Notes Section	Individualization of notebook; help dyads identify information to be kept in personal notes section (e.g., pill schedule, medical history, birthday list, bus schedule and maps, photos); develop pages.
Personal Goals	Discuss both fun (e.g., writing autobiography) and practical (e.g., planning for the future) personal goals; explore emotions and minimize issues that may cause problems reaching goals; identify ways to use the notebook to aid in completion of goals.

Despite the small sample size, all five very mild dementia participants endorsed feeling more confident that they could get support from family members and friends post-treatment (Coping Self Efficacy scale; Chesney, Neilands, Chambers, Taylor, and Folkman, 2006). In addition, all four coaches endorsed fewer symptoms of depression at post-treatment (Depression, Anxiety and Stress Scale; Lovibond and Lovibond, 1995). Notably, neither the participants nor the coaches reported higher levels of distress following the intervention, an important concern given past research reporting decreased patient morale and increased caregiver depression possibly resulting from greater awareness of impairment (Quayhagen, et al, 2000; Rabins, 1996). Modification of a standardized memory test (Rivermead Behavioral Memory Test- II; Wilson, Cockburn, and Baddeley, 2003), which allowed the early-stage dementia participants to take notes during memory testing, revealed significant improvement in participants' profile scores from pre-treatment to post-treatment. This improvement resulted from the early-stage dementia participants taking a greater amount of notes during learning, as well as remembering to reference those notes more often during delayed memory testing. These skills were stressed within the memory notebook training and suggest some generalization of the note taking skills. Unlike with the case study described earlier, despite a documented significant increase in use of the notebook and other memory strategies in the everyday lives of the early-stage dementia participants post-treatment, we were unable to show that these strategies decreased everyday memory lapses or resulted in improvement of functional independence for the care recipient in everyday life. During the course of treatment, there were no significant changes in the overall cognitive status of the early-stage dementia participants as documented by performances on tests that assessed premorbid intellectual abilities (North American Adult Reading Test; Blair and Spreen, 1989) and overall cognitive status (Repeatable Battery for Assessment of Neuropsychological Status; Randolph, Tierney, Mohr, and Chase, 1998).

The failure to find a significant impact of the intervention on everyday memory lapses or functional independence might reflect lack of sensitivity in the measures used or the group nature of the intervention. In comparison to the single-dyad format, the group format resulted in less time being devoted to individually tailoring the assignments and notebook use to each dyad's everyday living situation. On the other hand, a post-treatment focus group revealed a powerful effect of the group format on its members. The study participants indicated that they derived much comfort from knowing that they had a safe place where they could express themselves, talk (and at times laugh) about their difficulties and receive support from one another. As an example, during the application phase of the intervention, the group discussed end of life preparations; a topic that many had not openly discussed before. Group members reported that they were aware that these preparations needed to be discussed but were unsure about how to begin the discussion with their partners and family members. The group was able to problem-solve ways to start these discussions. The impact of this group support is further underscored by the fact that the group has continued to meet on their own for coffee once a month. This is reminiscent to what is often experienced with multiple family group treatment. The multiple family group format, which has been used in the schizophrenia and traumatic brain injury literatures (e.g., McFarlane, et al., 1995; Rogers, Norell, Short, Dyck, and Becker, 2007), has been shown to provide participants with an expanded informal support network, an empathic understanding of shared experiences, and information exchange on resources.

Conclusion

While the above findings suggest promise to blending cognitive rehabilitation with a dyadic intervention aimed at strengthening the relationship between the individual with early-stage dementia and the caregiver, there are limitations to the generalization of the study findings that must be carefully considered. First, although the very mild dementia participants and their coaches represented a diverse group in terms of age (range in age = 61-85), life experience, and occupation, they were all highly educated (16+ years of education). Second, all of the very mild dementia participants were aware that they were experiencing memory problems and were motivated and interested in learning methods to help compensate for their difficulties. Third, with the exception of memory, the remaining cognitive skills of all very mild dementia participants were generally well intact, thus helping to ensure that dementia participants would be able to successfully learn how to use the memory notebook. In teaching use of a memory notebook there is consensus that the memory impaired individual needs to be aware of their memory difficulties, trained to write clear information in the notebook and remain motivated to use the notebook on a consistent basis. The memory impaired individual also needs to receive extensive supervised practice (Dougherty and Radomski, 1987; Mateer and Sohlberg, 1988). As the benefits of memory notebook training are more apparent after high amounts of time have been invested into the training (e.g., after the notebook is set up and skills are cemented), it is important that both members of the care dyad continue to foster motivation and persistence throughout treatment.

As alluded to earlier, the group format appeared to be an important treatment factor at a variety of different levels. For example, it allowed group members access to other people's experiences and coping strategies as they attempted to deal with the effects of memory loss. Group members were also able to openly discuss difficulties and because they were at different stages in coping with the effects of memory loss, they could simultaneously guide and be guided by others in the group. Furthermore, group members were able to support each other and offer suggestions when faced with problems regarding memory notebook implementation. The group format also gave participants another avenue for increased social support. Despite the myriad of positive effects derived from the group format, one important challenge was the different learning speeds of the individuals. Although assigning each care dyad an individual therapist did help prevent participants from "being left behind" in the group, it may be helpful for future groups to consider ways to provide additional aid to individuals who end up struggling to acquire a specific skill, perhaps by scheduling one-on-one time with the dyad.

Scheduling the group to meet twice per week was an important factor in making the memory notebook an integral part of the group members' daily lives. However, at the conclusion of the 7-week intervention, we felt that the early-stage dementia participants would have benefited from additional practice and instruction (e.g., especially increased time spent writing in the memory notebook during treatment sessions), and that 20-24 training sessions might be a more appropriate target for future work. Other changes to the delivery of the intervention that may prove to be important in future work include maintaining a slower teaching pace, paying greater attention to integrating the memory notebook with systems already in place in the household, and simplifying the notebook sections. Although the majority of the intervention concentrated on teaching participants how to use the daily log section of the memory notebook to aid with retrospective and prospective memory failures, participants were also taught how to cross reference information with other sections of the notebook and to use the notebook calendar. These skills appeared less relevant to the everyday needs of most dyads. For example, all dyads already maintained a large joint wall calendar. Simplification of the memory notebook to the daily log section and a personal notes section (e.g., medication schedule, personal information etc.) may prove more beneficial for most dyads, with additional sections added as needed when relevant to the everyday lives of the care dyad.

We chose to utilize a large notebook (8 ½" X 12") and a timer with large numbers and a very loud alarm. We initially asked participants to have the alarm go off every hour to aid them in development of an over learned habit of regularly writing in the memory notebook. Although these considerations were practical and well thought out, they were met with some resistance by participants. Participants reported, for example, that the notebook was too large to fit in a purse and that the timer was too heavy, too loud, embarrassing, and went off at inconvenient times. Often participants did not want to take the large notebook with them on outings. One solution to this employed by several group members was to use sticky notes on outings and then to place them into the notebook. The general strategy of the intervention was to initially train participants with a standardized homogenous memory notebook, which could later be altered to better fit each care dyads needs. In future work, it may be more beneficial for the dyads to begin individualizing their notebooks from the beginning of training, thus creating a system that is personalized and fits the dyads current needs and goals. Future studies may want to allow for flexibility in choice of size of the memory notebook, and may also want to consider alternate methods for aiding participants in developing an over learned habit of regularly using the memory notebook. One useful strategy reported by our participants was writing in the notebook upon completion of an activity. In addition, future studies may want to help participants re-conceptualize the notebook from something that represents their disease process (and is embarrassing) to something that helps them plan for the future and remember the past.

One important facet of the intervention was the role of the coach (caregiver) in the memory notebook process. One of the challenges faced in the group was the seemingly diverse roles that the coaches took. Some coaches found it difficult to find a balance between helping too much and not helping enough. An important topic of discussion was how to be helpful without taking away their partner's power. Future studies should more fully explore the role of the coach. This might entail pre-group coach training in terms of identifying the most effective coaching style for facilitating memory notebook use, as well as how to incorporate this style into individual couple dynamics (e.g., how to encourage without "nagging"). In addition, it will be important to explore the couple's already existing complex dyadic relationship as a potential predictor of participant-coach interaction. Given the important role of familial support, the design of the intervention might also be improved by increasing the amount of time spent addressing communication and relationship issues. Devoting parts of some sessions to separately working with the coaches and participants may also prove useful. Initially we had planned to reserve time for the coaches and very mild dementia participants to meet separately. While the coaches seemed to appreciate this time, some of the very mild dementia participants expressed discomfort, feeling like they were being talked about. As this may prove to be an important component, future studies should consider ways of employing this brief separation in a way that is seen as mutually beneficially for both members of the care dyad.

To increase the impact of the intervention on the very mild dementia participants' everyday functioning, additional time spent better integrating use of the memory notebook into the dyads everyday lives would also likely prove beneficial. Although we had four therapists, each of whom were individually assigned to and responsible for a maximum of two dyads throughout treatment in order to provide individual assistance as needed, the pace of the intervention and number of sessions involved made it difficult to spend significant portions of time trying to personalize the memory notebook to the dyad's everyday life. Additional sessions and simplification of the memory notebook as discussed earlier would likely provide for more opportunities to better integrate the notebook so that it addresses specific needs in the everyday lives of the dyads. Future research will also be needed to determine whether this type of dyadic cognitive rehabilitative intervention can aid the psychological, social, emotional and economic costs associated with AD as the disease progresses. It was noted that by actively participating in memory notebook treatment, participants appeared to be reclaiming some control over the effects of memory loss. More specifically, participants seemed empowered by the decision to take back control by attending the group (e.g., "I am doing something in the face of this hardship"). In addition, participants learned how to use a memory notebook and acquired specific skills to help reduce the impact of memory loss (e.g., being able to determine what occurred yesterday without relying on others). Thus the intervention may have worked as both a symbolic and practical tool to minimize loss of control associated with memory problems.

Currently, the majority of behavioral treatment interventions for AD involve either treating only the AD patients or providing caregiver support and education separately from the care recipients. Given the intact awareness and higher cognitive skill levels of most early-stage dementia patients, interventions that include both members of the care dyad may represent a more optimal approach (Whitlatch, et al., 2006). Such an approach offers the potential to attend to the needs of both partners and to maintain the dyadic relationship through dealing more effectively with adjustments presented by memory impairments and behavioral deficits associated with AD. Moreover, most individuals with very mild dementia want to be proactive and demonstrate the ability for new learning, with non-drug therapies increasingly being recommended in conjunction with drug therapies to help improve/maintain everyday functioning (e.g., Koontz and Baskys, 2005; Seltzer, et al., 2004; De Vreese, et al., 2001). This further underscores the increasing need for a clear evidence base for cognitive rehabilitation in the treatment of very mild dementia (Clare and Woods, 2004). The results from the work presented suggest that blending a dyadic intervention with cognitive rehabilitation has the potential to facilitate adjustment and adaptation to the changes of dementia for both members of the care dyad while also maintaining hope and promoting functional independence.

References

Acevedo, A. and Loewenstein, D.A. (2007). Nonpharmacological cognitive interventions in aging and dementia. *Journal of Geriatric Psychiatry and Neurology*, *20*, 239-249.

Akkerman, R. L., and Ostwald, S. K. (2004). Reducing anxiety in Alzheimer's disease family caregivers: The effectiveness of a nine-week cognitive-behavioral intervention. *American Journal of Alzheimer's Disease and Other Dementias*, *19*, 117-123.

American Psychiatric Association (1997). Practice guidelines. Workgroup on Alzheimer's disease and related disorders. In *Practice Guideline for the Treatment of Patients with Alzheimer's Disease and Other Dementias*, Rabins (Ed.). The American Journal of Psychiatry, 154s, 1-39.

Baines, S., Saxby, P. and Ehlert, K. (1987). Reality orientation and reminiscence therapy: A controlled cross-over study of elderly confused people. *British Journal of Psychiatry*, *151*, 222-231.

Ballard, C. G., Bannister, V., Oyebode, F. (1996). Depression in dementia sufferers. *International Journal of Geriatric Psychiatry*, *11*, 987-990.

Ballard, C. G., Boyle, A., Bowler, C., and Lindesay, J. (1996). Anxiety disorders in dementia sufferers. *International Journal of Geriatric Psychiatry*, *11*, 507-515.

Berger, G., Bernhardt, T., Schramm, U., Müller, R., Landsiedel-Anders, S., Peters, J., et al. (2004). No effects of a combination of caregivers support group and memory training/music therapy in dementia patients from a memory clinic population. *International Journal of Geriatric Psychiatry*, *19*, 223-231.

Berry, E., Kapur, N., Williams, L., Hodges, S., Watson, P., Smyth, Get al. (2007). The use of a wearable camera, SenseCam, as a pictorial diary to improve autobiographical memory in patient with limbic encephalitis: A preliminary report. *Neuropsychological Rehabilitation*, *17*, 582-601.

Blair, J.R. and Spreen, O. (1989). Predicting premorbid IQ: A revision of the National Adult Reading Test. *Clinical Neuropsychologist*, *3*, 129-136.

Brodaty, H. (2007). Meaning and measurement of caregiver outcomes. *International Psychogeriatrics. Special Issue: Focus on defining and measuring treatment benefits in dementia*, *19(3)*, 363-381.

Bourgeois, M.S., Camp, C., Rose, M., White, B., Malone, M., Carr, J., et al. (2003). A comparison of training strategies to enhance use of external aids by persons with dementia. *Journal of Communication Disorders*, *36*, 361-378.

Cahn-Weiner, D.A., Malloy, P.F., Rebok, G.W., and Ott, B.R. (2003). Results of a randomized placebo-controlled study of memory training for mildly impaired Alzheimer's disease patients. *Applied Neuropsychology*, *10*, 215-223.

Camp, C.J., Foss, J.W., O'Hanlon, A.M., and Stevens, A.B. (1996). Memory interventions for persons with dementia. *Applied Cognitive Psychology*, *10*, 193-210.

Camp, C.J., Foss, J.W., Stevens, A.B., O'Hanlon, A.M., Brandimonte, M., Einstein, G.O., et al. (1996). Improving prospective memory task performance in persons with Alzheimer's disease. In *Prospective memory: Theory and applications* (pp. 351-367). Mahwah, NJ, US: Lawrence Erlbaum Associates Publishers.

Chesney, M.A., Neilands, T.B., Chambers, D.B., Taylor, J.M., and Folkman, S. (2006). A validity and reliability study of the Coping Self-Efficacy scale. *British Journal of Health Psychology, 11*, 421-437.

Clare, L. (2002). Developing awareness about awareness in early-stage dementia: The role of psychosocial factors. *Dementia: The International Journal of Social Research and Practice, 1*, 295-312.

Clare, L., Wilson, B.A., Breen, K., and Hodges, J.R. (1999). Errorless learning of face-name associations in early Alzheimer's disease. *Neurocase,* 5(1), 37-46.

Clare, L., Wilson, B.A., Carter, G., Breen, K., Gosses, A., and Hodges, J.R. (2000). Intervening with everyday memory problems in dementia of Alzheimer type: An errorless learning approach. *Journal of Clinical and Experimental Neuropsychology, 22*, 132-146.

Clare, L., and Woods, R. T. (2004). Cognitive training and cognitive rehabilitation for people with early-stage Alzheimer's disease: A review. *Neuropsychological Rehabilitation, 14*, 385-401.

Coon, D.W., Thompson, L., Steffen, A., Sorocco, K., and Gallagher-Thompson, D. (2003). Anger and Depression Management: Psychoeducational Skill Training Interventions for Women Caregivers of a Relative With Dementia. *The Gerontologist, 43*, 678-689.

Corbeil, R.R., Quayhagen, M.P., and Quayhagen, M. (1999). Intervention effects on dementia caregiving interaction: A stress-adaptation modeling approach. *Journal of Aging and Health, 11*, 79-95.

Derogatis, L. R. (1975). *SCL-90: Administration, scoring, and procedures manual, I, for the R version*. Baltimore, John Hopkins University School of Medicine.

De Vreese, L.P., Neri, M., Fioravanti, M., Belloi, L., and Zanetti, O. (2001). Memory rehabilitation in Alzheimer's disease: A review of progress. *International Journal of Geriatric Psychiatry, 16*, 794-809.

Dougherty, P. M., and Radomski, M. V. (1987). *The cognitive rehabilitation workbook.* Salem: Aspen Publishers Inc.

Epstein, C., Auclair, U., and Mittelman, M. (2007). Couples Counseling in Alzheimer's Disease: First Observations of a Novel Intervention Study. *Clinical Gerontologist, 30*, 21-35.

Farias, S.T., Mungas, D., Reed, B.R., Harvey, D., Cahn-Weiner, D., and DeCarli, C. (2006). MCI is Associated With Deficits in Everyday Functioning. *Alzheimer Disease and Associated Disorders, 20*, 217-223.

Farina, E., Fioravanti, R., Chiavari, L., Imbornone, E., Alberoni, M., Pomati, S., et al. (2002). Comparing two programs of cognitive training in Alzheimer's disease: A pilot study. *Acta Neurologica Scandinavica, 105*, 365-371.

Folstein, M.F., Folstein, S.E., and McHugh, P.R. (1975). Mini-mental state: A practical method for grading the cognitive state of patients for the clinician. *Journal of Psychiatric Research, 12*, 189-198.

Goldsilver, P. M., and Gruneir, M. R. (2001). Early stage dementia group: An innovative model of support for individuals in the early stages of dementia. *American Journal of Alzheimer's Disease and Other Dementias, 16*, 109-114.

Hebert, L.E., Scherr, P. A., Bienias, J. L., Bennett, D. A., and Evans, D. A. (2003). Alzheimer Disease in the U.S. Population: Prevalence Estimates Using the 2000 Census. *Archives of Neurology, 60*, 1119–1122.

Holmes, T. (2000). Use of a memory notebook to help Alzheimer caregivers manage behavioral excesses. *Physical and Occupational Therapy in Geriatrics, 17*, 67-80.

Hughes, C. P., Berg, L., Danzinger, W. L., Coben, L. A., and Martin, R. L. (1982). A new clinical scale for the staging of dementia. *British Journal of Psychiatry, 140*, 566-572.

Koontz, J. and Baskys, A. (2005). Effects of galantamine on working memory and global functioning in patients with mild cognitive impairment: A double-blind placebo-controlled study. *American Journal of Alzheimer's Disease and Other Dementias, 20*, 295-302.

Langill, M., and Schmitter-Edgecombe, M. (May, 2007). *Memory notebook training for very mild dementia: A case study*. Presented at the 33rd annual meeting of the ABA, San Diego, CA.

Lewin Group (2004). *Saving Lives, Saving Money: Dividends for Americans Investing in Alzheimer Research.* A report commissioned by the Alzheimer's Association. Washington (DC): The Lewin Group.

Loewenstein, D.A., Acevedo, A., Czaja, S.J., and Duara, R. (2004). Cognitive rehabilitation of mildly impaired Alzheimer disease patients on cholinesterase inhibitors. *American Journal of Geriatric Psychiatry, 12*, 395-402.

Logsdon, R.G., McCurry, S.M., and Teri, L. (2007). Evidence-based psychological treatments for disruptive behaviors in individuals with dementia. *Psychology and Aging, 22*, 28-36.

Lovibond, S. H., and Lovibond, P. F. (1995) *Manual for the Depression Anxiety Stress Scales (2nd. Ed.).* Sydney: Psychology Foundation.

Maeda, K. (2005). Editorial: Cognitive rehabilitation for Alzheimer's disease. *Psychogeriatrics, 5*, 1-2.

Marriott, A., Donaldson, C., Tarrier, N., and Burns, A. (2000). Effectiveness of cognitive-behavioural family intervention in reducing the burden of care in carers of patients with Alzheimer's disease. *British Journal of Psychiatry, 176*, 557-562.

Mateer, C. A., and Sohlberg, M. M. (1988). A paradigm shift in memory rehabilitation. In H. Whitaker (Ed)., *Neuropsychological studies of non-focal brain damage: Dementia and trauma* (pp. 202-225). New York: Springer-Verlag.

McFarlane, W.R., Lukens, E., Link, B., Dushay, R., Deakins, S. A., Newmark, M., et al. (1995). Multiple-family groups and psychoeducation in the treatment of schizophrenia. *Archives of General Psychiatry, 52*, 679-687.

Morris, J. C. (1993). The Clinical Dementia Rating (CDR): Current version and scoring rules. *Neurology, 43*, 2412-2414.

Morris, J. C., McKeel, D. W., Storandt, M., Rubin, E. H., Price, J. L., Grant, E. A., et al. (1991).Very mild Alzheimer's disease: informant-based clinical, psychometric, and pathologic distinction from normal aging. *Neurology, 41*, 469-478.

Onor, M.L., Trevisiol, M., Negro, C., Alessandra, S., Saina, M., and Aguglia, E. (2007). Impact of a multimodal rehabilitative intervention on demented patients and their caregivers. *American Journal of Alzheimer's Disease and Other Dementias, 22*, 261-272.

Quayhagen, M.P., and Quayhagen, M. (2001). Testing of a cognitive stimulation intervention for dementia caregiving dyads. *Neuropsychological Rehabilitation, 11*, 319-332.

Quayhagen, M.P., Quayhagen, M., Corbeil, R.R., Hendrix, R.C., Jackson, J.E., Snyder, L., et al. (2000). Coping with dementia: Evaluation of four non pharmacologic interventions. *International Psychogeriatrics, 12*, 249-265.

Quayhagen, M., Quayhagen, M., Corbeil, R.R., Roth, P.A., and Rogers, J. A. (1995). A dyadic remediation program for care recipients with dementia. *Nursing Research, 44*, 153-159.

Quittre, A., Oliver, C., and Salmon, E. (2005). Compensating strategies for impaired episodic memory and time orientation in a patient with Alzheimer's disease. *Acta Neurologica Belgica, 105*, 30-38.

Rabins, P. V. (1996). Developing treatment guidelines for Alzheimer's disease and other dementias. *Journal of Clinical Psychiatry, 57*, 37-38.

Randolph, C., Tierney, M.C., Mohr, E., and Chase, T.N. (1998). The Repeatable Battery for the Assessment of Neuropsychological Status (RBANS): Preliminary clinical validity. *Journal of Clinical and Experimental Neuropsychology, 20*, 310-319.

Requena, C., López lbor, M. I., Maestú, F., Campo, P., López lbor, J. J., and Ortiz, T. (2004). Effects of Cholinergic Drugs and Cognitive Training on Dementia. *Dementia and Geriatric Cognitive Disorders, 18*, 50-54.

Rogers, M.L., Norell, D.M., Short, R.A., Dyck, D., and Becker, B. (2007). Adapting multi-family group treatment for brain and spinal cord injury. *Am. J. Phys. Med. Rehab., 86*, 482-492.

Schmitter-Edgecombe, M., Fahy, J. F., Whelan, J. P., and Long, C. J. (1995). Memory remediation after severe closed-head injury: Notebook training versus supportive therapy. *Journal of Consulting and Clinical Psychology, 63,* 484-489

Schmitter-Edgecombe, M., Howard, J. T., Pavawalla, S., Howell, L. and Rueda, A. (submitted). *Multi-dyad Memory Notebook Intervention for Very Mild Dementia: A Pilot Study.*

Seltzer, B., Zolnouni, P., Nunez, M., Goldman, R., Kumar, D., Ieni, J., et al. (2004). Efficacy of Donepezil in Early-Stage Alzheimer Disease: A Randomized Placebo-Controlled Trial. *Archives of Neurology, 61*, 1852-1856.

Smits, C. H. M., de Lange, J., Dröes, R. M., Meiland, F., Vernooij-Dassen, M. , and Pot, A. M. (2007). Effects of combined intervention programs for people with dementia living at home and their caregivers: A systematic review. *International Journal of Geriatric Psychiatry, 22*, 1181-1193.

Sohlberg, M.M., and Mateer, C.A. (1989). Training use of compensatory memory books: A three stage behavioral approach. *Journal of Clinical and Experimental Neuropsychology, 11*, 871-891.

Steffen, A.M. and Berger, S. (2000). Relationship differences in anger intensity during caregiving-related situations. *Clinical Gerontologist, 21*, 3-19.

Teri, L., Logsdon, R.G., Uomoto, J., and McCurry, S.M. (1997). Behavioral treatment of depression in dementia patients: A controlled clinical trial. *Journals of Gerontology: Series B: Psychological Sciences and Social Sciences, 52B*, 159-166.

Unverzagt, F.W., Kasten, L., Johnson, K.E., Rebok, G.W., Marsiske, M., Koepke, K.M., et al. (2007). Effect of memory impairment on training outcomes in ACTIVE. *Journal of the International Neuropsychological Society, 13*, 953-960.

Vitaliano, P., Echeverria, D., Shelkey, M., Zhang, J., and Scanlan, J. (2007). A cognitive psychophysiological model to predict functional decline in chronically stressed older adults. *Journal of Clinical Psychological Medicine, 14*, 177-190.

Whitlatch, C. J., Judge, K., Zarit, S. H., and Femia, E. (2006). Dyadic intervention for family caregivers and care receivers in early-stage dementia. *The Gerontologist, 46*, 688-694.

Wilson, B.A., Cockburn, J., and Baddeley, A. (2003). *The Rivermead Behavioural Memory Test,* 2nd edition (RBMT-II). UK: Thames Valley Test Co.

Yesavage, J. A., Brink, T. L., Rose, T. L., Lum, O., Huang, V. Adey, M. B., et al. (1983). Development and validation of a geriatric depression rating scale: A preliminary report. *Journal of Psychiatric Research, 17*, 37-49.

Zarit, S.H., and Edwards, A.B. (1996). Family caregiving: Research and clinical intervention. In R.T. Woods (Ed.), *Handbook of the clinical psychology of ageing* (pp. 331-368). Oxford, England: John Wiley and Sons.

Zarit, S.H., Femia, E.E., Watson, J., Rice-Oeschger, L., and Kakos, B. (2004). Memory club: A group intervention for people with early-stage dementia and their care partners. *The Gerontologist, 44*, 262-269.

Zarit, S.H. and Leitsch, S.A. (2001). Developing and evaluating community based intervention programs for Alzheimer's patients and their caregivers. *Aging and Mental Health, 5*, 84-98.

In: New Directions in Aging Research
Editor: Ruby R. Brougham, pp. 57-73

ISBN 978-1-60741-976-1
© 2009 Nova Science Publishers, Inc.

Chapter 4

Living Well with MCI: Behavioral Interventions for Older Adults with Mild Cognitive Impairment

Adriana M. Seelye**, Diane B. Howieson, Katherine V. Wild, Luis R. Sauceda and Jeffrey A. Kaye

Oregon Health and Science University, Department of Neurology, Portland, Oregon, USA

Abstract

Along with identifying effective medications, the development and evaluation of behavioral interventions to assist in managing symptoms and improving quality of life in persons with MCI is critical. In this chapter, we first review the literature on behavioral interventions used with healthy older adults and individuals with MCI and AD. We then report on a pilot study from our research group that examined the feasibility of two behavioral interventions to improve daily function and quality of life in individuals with MCI. One intervention used electronic memory devices to compensate for memory impairment and the other intervention used cognitive-behavioral therapy techniques and training with non-electronic memory aids. Challenges associated with implementing a behavioral intervention for MCI patients are discussed, along with recommendations for establishing an MCI treatment program. Further development and validation of behavioral interventions that could be accessible to and employed by clinics and hospitals where MCI patients receive diagnosis and treatment are needed.

* Correspondence should be addressed to Adriana M. Seelye, Department of Psychology, Washington State University, Pullman, Washington 99164-4820. Phone: 509-592-3324. FAX: 509-335-5043. Electronic mail may be sent to aseelye@wsu.edu

Introduction

Attention to the early stages of development of Alzheimer's disease (AD) has increased in recent years. MCI indicates that an individual has a decline in memory greater than expected for age but the degree of cognitive impairment does not fulfill diagnostic criteria for dementia (Winblad, et al, 2004). Recent studies have demonstrated that MCI is associated with impairments in daily functioning, particularly those activities dependent on memory (Farias, et al, 2006; Wadley, et al., 2007). As the general population ages the number of elderly individuals diagnosed with MCI is increasing. In a study of cognitive decline in the elderly, 34% of MCI patients developed AD within five years, a rate much higher than in individuals without MCI (Bennett, et al., 2002). In the oldest old population, the progression to AD in MCI patients is even greater, 56% in five years in our study (Howieson, et al., 2003).

The increasing number of individuals with MCI is a growing public health concern, since the decline in function and independence associated with MCI can be personally and financially devastating for patients, caregivers, and the public. Along with identifying effective medications, the development and evaluation of behavioral interventions to assist in managing symptoms and improving quality of life in persons with MCI is critical. These individuals may lose independence as concerned family members insist that they be supervised. However, many individuals with MCI are eager to learn ways to manage their memory difficulties and maintain their independence. With the aging of the U.S. population, the number of individuals with MCI seeking assistance with memory problems, independence, and daily functioning, is bound to grow.

We begin this chapter with a brief review of behavioral interventions that have been used with healthy older adults, and patients with MCI and AD. Specifically, we discuss evidence for the utility of cognitive therapy techniques, non-electronic and electronic external memory aids, and errorless learning approaches as components of behavioral interventions. We then report on pilot work from our research group that examined the feasibility of two behavioral interventions to improve daily function and quality of life in individuals with MCI. One intervention used electronic memory devices to compensate for memory impairment and the other intervention used cognitive-behavioral therapy techniques and training with non-electronic memory aids. In the last section, we discuss challenges and successes associated with implementing these types of behavioral interventions for MCI patients, along with recommendations for establishing an MCI treatment program.

Cognitive Training Programs

Cognitive training programs have been shown to improve cognitive functioning (Ball, et al., 2002; Mohs, et al., 1998; Singer, Lindenberger, and Baltes, 2003) and subjective memory appraisal (Floyd and Scogin, 1997; Lachman, Weaver, Bandura, Elliott, and Lewkowicz, 1992) in healthy elderly. However, cognitive rehabilitation training in patients with MCI and early AD has yielded mixed results (Backman, Josephsson, Herlitz, Stigsdotter, and Viitanen, 1991; Belleville, et al., 2006; Onor, et al., 2007). While MCI patients' memory performances have been shown to improve with some forms of cognitive training (Belleville, et al., 2006), their memory performances have not improved in other studies (Onor, et al., 2007; Rapp, Brenes, and Marsh, 2002). The benefits of cognitive training with AD patients have been more effective in some cognitive domains than others (Sitzer, Twamley, and Jeste, 2006 for a review; Talassi, et al., 2007). Disappointingly, however, improvements in Alzheimer patients' performances on specific cognitive tasks do not necessarily generalize to unrelated, novel situations (Loewenstein, Acevedo, Czaja, and Dura, 2004). AD patients may benefit less than MCI patients from cognitive training because their memory impairment is more severe and because they would be expected to have weaker potential for use of cognitive strategies.

Rapp, et al. (2002) examined the effectiveness of cognitive training for individuals with MCI. Although memory training did not improve objective memory performance, cognitive therapy techniques such as cognitive restructuring improved participants' perceived memory abilities and feelings of control over memory. Given that perceived memory abilities and memory control beliefs have been associated with improved memory functioning on real-world tasks (Mohs, et al., 1998) and increased motivation and self-efficacy (Rapp, et al., 2002), further research focused in this area is warranted.

Although both MCI and mild AD elders have memory problems, those with MCI may have better cognitive resources for developing memory compensation strategies. One strategy for helping MCI patients cope with memory problems is the use of external memory aids. Patients with MCI (Greenaway, et al., 2006) and very mild dementia (Schmitter-Edgecombe, Howard, Pavawalla, Howell, and Rueda, in press) can learn to use and benefit from memory notebook training to compensate for memory loss. In these studies, MCI patients reported increased self-efficacy, improved daily functioning (Greenaway, et al., 2006), increased use of memory compensation strategies, and increased confidence in their ability to obtain support from family members (Schmitter-Edgecombe, et al., in press) following memory notebook training.

Training in the use of electronic devices has been used to help patients with traumatic brain injuries compensate for memory loss. Electronic devices used include voice organizers, voice recorders, pagers, and electronic reminders (Hart, Buchhofer, and Vaccaro, 2004; O'Neil-Pirozzi, Kendrick, Goldstein, and Glenn, 2004; van den Broek, Downes, Johnson, Dayus, and Hilton, 2000). In one of the few studies that examined the use of electronic memory aids for Alzheimer patients, participants benefited more from using an electronic device than using written reminders or no assistance at all (Oriani, et al., 2003). No studies known to us have examined the feasibility of training MCI patients to use electronic memory aids to compensate for memory loss.

Specific instructional techniques such as errorless learning have proved successful in teaching new information to individuals with developmental disabilities (Sohlberg, Ehlhardt, and Kennedy, 2005), traumatic brain injuries, and AD (Clare, et al., 2000; Mimura, and Komatsu, 2007). Errorless learning is designed to reduce errors during the acquisition phase of learning by breaking tasks down into small steps, modeling the correct behavior for the learner in advance, discouraging guessing, immediately correcting errors, and fading prompts (Sohlberg, Ehlhardt, and Kennedy, 2005). Errorless learning techniques can be applied to various every day tasks and may improve independence and quality of life (Wilson, Baddeley, Evans, and Shiel, 1994).

Our pilot study examined the feasibility of two multifaceted behavioral interventions to improve daily function and quality of life in individuals with MCI. The cognitive-behavioral therapy (CBT) intervention included training with non- electronic memory aids through errorless learning instruction in addition to cognitive-behavioral therapy techniques and strategies to manage emotional reactions to improve subjective memory appraisal and perceived control over memory. The electronic memory device (EMD) intervention included training with electronic memory aids through errorless learning training and supervised rehearsal to compensate for memory impairment. It was hypothesized that following training, participants in both groups would report improvement in daily functioning, mood, quality of life, and increased use of memory compensation strategies, although they would not show improvement on objective memory testing. Furthermore, it was hypothesized that participants in the CBT group would report improvement in perceived control over memory and subjective memory appraisal. The main purpose of this pilot study was to explore ways to assist MCI patients in compensating for memory problems.

Method

Participants

Participant pairs in the present study were community-dwelling, older adults classified as having MCI based on their most recent evaluation by a neurologist in one of two Alzheimer clinics (n = 16) or by telephone interview with a brief memory examination (Loewenstein, et al., 2000) (n = 2) and their representatives, referred to as "study partners." Of the 18 participants recruited into the program, six participants were assigned to the CBT group, six participants were assigned to the EMD group, and six participants were assigned to the wait-list control group. Two participants and their study partners dropped out of the program. One participant dropped out of the EMD group after the second session because of significant health problems. The other participant dropped out of the CBT group after the fourth session and did not report the reason. Of the six participants recruited into the wait-list control group, three were assigned to the CBT group and three were assigned to the EMD group. Table 1 shows participant characteristics by group at entry. Participants who completed the program included 9 women and 7 men. Fourteen participants were married, one was divorced, and one was widowed. Fifteen participants identified as Caucasian and one did not answer. Participants' education levels ranged from 12-20 years.

Prospective participants were excluded if they had a diagnosis of dementia or other cognitive disorder; had a diagnosis of a major psychiatric disorder; lacked insight into their memory problems; were unable to function independently with little to no difficulty in their daily activities; were unable to commit to attending weekly 1-hour sessions for an 11-week intervention program; were unable to secure reliable transportation to and from weekly sessions; or did not have a study partner.

Table 1. Participant characteristics by group at entry and memory performance on the HVLT-R in t-scores

Variable	CBT (n = 9)	EMD (n = 9)	Wait-list Control (n = 6)
Age M(SD)	71.60 (5.86)	74.94 (8.85)	74.10 (8.54)
Gender (%)			
Male	56	33	33
Female	44	67	67
Marital status (%)			
Married	100	78	83
Divorced		11	
Widowed		11	17
Education M(SD)	15.67 (2.18)	15.83 (1.94)	15.17 (1.60)
Ethnicity (%)			
Caucasian	100	89	100
No answer		11	
Memory Performance M(SD)			
HVLT-R Total Recall	40.11 (9.97)	36.67 (12.69)	43.17 (10.78)
HVLT-R Delay Recall	34.22 (17.56)	34.33 (12.59)	41.00 (12.57)
HVLT-R Discrimination Index	34.50 (12.80)	30.89 (13.86)	40.33 (10.86)

Note. After being wait-listed, the six control participants were assigned evenly to the CBT and EMD intervention groups.

Study partners attended the program and assisted with implementation of the program and "home exercises." Study partners were spouses except for three cases; two were friends and one was a daughter living separately.

Measures

Daily Functioning. A modified version of the Community Integration Questionnaire (CIQ; Willer, Rosenthal, Kreutzer, Gordon, and Rempel, 1993) was used to assess functional status of participants. The CIQ contains 15 items that comprise three subscales: home integration, social integration, and productive activities. The Functional Activities Questionnaire (FAQ; Pfeffer, Kurosaki, Harrah, Chance, and Filos, 1982) was used in assessing study partners perceptions of participants' functional abilities. Study partners rated the participants' performance on 10 complex activities of daily living, with higher scores indicating higher dependence.

Quality of Life. The Quality of Life Enjoyment and Satisfaction Questionnaire, Short Form (QLESQ; Endicott, Nee, Harrison, and Blumenthal, 1993) is a self-report measure that was used to assess participants' quality of life. The QLESQ, Short Form contains 16 items that measure the amount of enjoyment and satisfaction experienced in general activities. Participants rated their satisfaction on a 5-point scale, with higher scores indicating higher quality of life.

Mood. The Geriatric Depression Scale (GDS; Yesavage, 1988) was used to assess participants' mood. The GDS contains 30 yes/no items that assess the presence or absence of depressive symptoms.

Memory Compensation Strategy Use. The Memory Compensation Questionnaire (MCQ; Dixon, De Frias, and Backman, 2001) was used to assess participants' reported use of memory compensation strategies. The MCQ contains 40 items that comprise five subscales of memory compensation behavior (External, Internal, Reliance, Time, and Effort). Participants rated the frequency of memory compensation strategy use on a five-point Likert scale, with higher scores indicating more frequent use of the memory compensation behavior.

Perceived Control over Memory. The Memory Controllability Inventory (MC Inventory; Lachman, Weaver, and Elliot, 1995) was used to assess participants' perceived control over memory and perceived memory ability. The MC Inventory contains 19 items that comprise six subscales (Present Ability, Potential Improvement, Effort Utility, Inevitable Decrement, Independence, and Alzheimer's Likelihood). Participants rated each item on a seven-point Likert scale, with higher scores indicating higher agreement.

Perceived Memory Ability. The Memory Functioning Questionnaire (MFQ; Zelinski, Gilewski, and Anthony-Bergstone, 1990) was used to assess participants' subjective appraisal of memory abilities. The MFQ contains 64 items that comprise four subscales, two of which were used: general frequency of forgetting (Frequency) and change relative to retrospective functioning (Retrospective). Participants rated each item on a seven-point Likert scale, with higher scores indicating less frequent memory problems. In addition, collaterals rated the frequency of their participants' memory problems.

Memory Performance. The Hopkins Verbal Memory Test- Revised (HVLT-R; Shapiro, Benedict, Schretlen, and Brandt, 1999) was used to assess participants' objective verbal memory performance. The HVLT-R consists of a brief 12-item word list with immediate recall, delayed recall, and recognition trials. Higher scores indicate better memory performance. The HVLT-R contains three equivalent alternate forms that were used for repeated assessments to minimize a practice effect.

Procedure

Individuals who met all study criteria were matched for age and assigned either to the CBT group, the EMD group, or to the wait-list control group. Full randomization was not possible because some participants could attend at only one of the time slots. However, these participants did not know which treatment intervention was associated with their desired time slot. To facilitate recruitment, two waves of recruitment and programs were conducted. Both waves 1 and 2 consisted of a CBT and EMD intervention. Each intervention consisted of eleven weekly group meetings lasting one hour that were attended by participants and their study partners and were facilitated by a neuropsychologist, a health psychologist, and two research assistants. Each session began with review and discussion of the past week's material. The majority of time was spent introducing new material, facilitators modeling and demonstrating new skills and techniques, participants and study partners practicing new skills and techniques, and facilitators providing feedback. Sessions concluded with the assignment of a "home exercise" for participants to practice using the skill or technique with the assistance of their study partners during the upcoming week. Participants were provided with the memory aids to use during the intervention and to keep after the study ended.

The first and last of the 11 meetings consisted of administration of outcome measures to participants and study partners. Both groups received didactic information followed by a general discussion at the second session. Topics covered included current memory problems, recommended physical, social, and leisure activities, changes in cognition associated with normal aging, and the nature and significance of an MCI diagnosis (See Appendix for an outline of session topics from wave 2 CBT and EMD interventions).

CBT condition. During the remaining sessions, facilitators discussed maladaptive and adaptive ways to view memory problems and role-played examples of overly negative, overly positive, and realistic responses to memory failures. An emphasis was placed on fostering participants' motivation to use external compensation strategies to cope more effectively with their memory problems. Additionally, internal techniques to improve memory were introduced as strategies to help participants remember information until they had the opportunity to transfer it to a permanent location. Organization, reliable systems of tracking information, keeping routines and habits, and setting realistic goals were discussed. Facilitators trained participants to use several non-electronic memory aids through errorless learning instruction, including a telephone message book, a dry erase whiteboard, and a non-electronic personal organizer that included a monthly calendar, weekly appointment schedule, and a daily "to-do" list. The training concluded with a review of program topics and an opportunity for participants and study partners to give feedback. Modifications were made to the wave 2 CBT intervention based on feedback from wave 1 participants, including one additional session focused on training participants to use the non-electronic personal organizer.

EMD condition. The first and second sessions were as similar to the CBT condition as possible. During the remaining sessions, facilitators trained participants to use internal memory techniques and used role-plays to demonstrate how to use internal memory techniques effectively. Facilitators trained participants to use several electronic memory aids through errorless learning instruction, including an electronic locating device and a digital voice recorder. Many participants and study partners reported having difficulty using the electronic memory aids, so modifications were made to the wave 2 EMD intervention based on feedback from wave 1, including training with simpler models of the electronic memory devices. Specific modifications included training with a different model electronic object finder, training with a microcassette voice recorder as an alternative to a digital voice recorder, and training with the calculator, world clock, note pad, and calendar functions of a simple electronic personal digital assistant (PDA), the Palm Z22.

Wait-List control condition. Participants in this group filled out all baseline outcome measures at entry and after 11 weeks with no intervention. These participants were then matched for age and randomly assigned to either the CBT or EMD group in Wave 2.

Follow-up. The wave 1 participants completed follow-up outcome measures three months and six months after the program while wave 2 participants completed follow-up outcome measures only at three months.

Results

T-tests and chi-square analyses compared groups at baseline on demographic variables. Paired t-tests evaluated treatment effects between pre- and post-test and pre- to 3- and 6-month follow-up. Unpaired t-tests compared participants and study partners ratings of participants' daily functioning and subjective memory appraisal at baseline and at the end of the intervention. Because of the exploratory nature of the study and small sample sizes, a significance level of .05 was accepted despite multiple comparisons.

There were no statistically significant differences between groups in age, gender, ethnicity, education, or HVLT-R scores at baseline.

Table 2 presents the group means and standard deviations only for outcome measures with statistically significant treatment effects at pre-test, post-test, or 3- and 6- month follow-up.

Table 2. Means and standard deviations for outcome measures by treatment condition on outcome measures where statistical differences were found

Treatment	Start Program M(SD)	End Program M(SD)	Follow-up 3 Months M(SD)	Follow-up 6 Months M(SD)
Participants				
CIQ- Home Subscale				
CBT	5.00 (2.59)	5.19 (3.09)	6.11 (2.88)	4.63 (1.44)
EMD	5.19 (3.02)	6.09 (2.36)*	5.80 (2.81)	6.27 (1.25)
Controls	5.41 (3.23)	5.26 (2.89)		
CIQ- Social Subscale				
CBT	8.25 (2.05)	7.87 (2.42)	8.75 (2.31)	7.67 (1.15)
EMD	9.37 (2.13)	8.87 (1.96)	9.25 (2.43)	8.33 (1.15)
Controls	9.33 (1.75)	9.5 (2.17)		
CIQ- Productivity Subscale				
CBT	3.87 (1.55)	3.63 (1.69)	3.25 (1.39)	4.00 (0.00)
EMD	3.13 (1.64)	3.38 (1.69)	2.75 (1.49)	4.33 (2.08)
Controls	2.67 (.81)	4.33 (1.97)		
CIQ- Total Score				
CBT	17.16 (3.44)	16.70 (3.92)	18.11 (3.02)	14.97 (0.28)
EMD	17.70 (5.43)	17.46 (4.86)	17.80 (5.00)	18.93 (1.60)
Controls	17.42 (3.82)	19.10 (3.50)		
MC Inventory- Present Ability Subscale				
CBT	3.62 (0.90)	4.75(1.12)**	4.00 (1.48)	4.78 (1.65)
EMD	3.00 (0.93)	3.79 (1.26)	3.62 (0.74)	2.78 (1.35)
Controls	3.55 (0.75)	4.22 (0.72)*		
MC Inventory- Potential for Improvement Subscale				
CBT	4.79 (1.15)	4.96 (1.04)	5.37 (0.95)	5.77 (0.69)
EMD	4.60 (1.30)	4.75 (0.99)	4.58 (0.94)	5.22 (0.19)
Controls	4.88 (1.07)	4.77 (1.38)		

Treatment	Start Program M(SD)	End Program M(SD)	Follow-up 3 Months M(SD)	Follow-up 6 Months M(SD)
MC Inventory- Effort Made Subscale				
CBT	5.50 (0.89)	5.16 (0.69)	5.37 (0.72)	5.78 (0.78)
EMD	4.95 (1.00)	4.75 (1.04)	4.21 (1.31)	3.89 (1.39)
Controls	4.55 (1.09)	5.27 (0.77)		
MC Inventory- Inevitable Decrement Subscale				
CBT	3.49 (0.89)	3.16 (0.99)	3.25 (1.42)	3.11 (0.70)
EMD	4.29 (1.40)	3.54 (1.54)	4.00 (1.17)	4. 45 (0.39)
Controls	3.55 (0.59)	3.66 (0.92)		
MC Inventory- Independence Subscale				
CBT	3.33 (0.69)	2.91 (0.64)	3.08 (1.07)	4.00 (0.67)
EMD	3.20 (1.04)	3.71 (1.33)	3.54 (1.63)	4.00 (1.00)
Controls	2.99 (0.56)	3.39 (0.68)		
MC Inventory- AD Likelihood Subscale				
CBT	4.15 (1.97)	4.12 (1.19)	4.31 (1.97)	4.67 (0.88)
EMD	4.12 (1.61)	4.46 (1.63)	4.50 (1.97)	3.50 (2.38)
Controls	5.16 (1.27)	4.87 (1.43)		
MC Inventory-Total Score				
CBT	24.90 (1.45)	25.08 (1.48)	25.41 (1.46)	27.80 (2.07)
EMD	24.18 (2.01)	25.01 (1.42)	24.48 (2.92)	23.17 (2.11)
Controls	24.71 (1.36)	25.31 (1.48)		
Study Partners				
CIQ- Home Subscale				
CBT	6.25 (2.17)	5.71 (2.69)	3.79 (3.15)	3.43 (2.97)
EMD	5.42 (3.03)	5.42 (3.03)	5.33 (3.11)	5.43 (1.89)
Controls	5.75 (3.01)	7.75 (1.05)		
CIQ- Social Subscale				
CBT	8.35 (3.30)	8.29 (3.25)	6.00 (3.83)	7.67 (2.51)
EMD	8.33 (2.42)	7.17 (2.32)	8.37 (2.77)	9.67 (0.58)
Controls	7.80 (2.59)	8.80 (2.59)		
CIQ- Productivity Subscale				
CBT	3.28 (1.60)	3.14 (2.19)	2.14 (2.67)	0.50 (0.71)
EMD	3.40 (1.52)	3.80 (2.28)	3.12 (1.36)	4.50 (0.71)
Controls	3.20 (1.10)	4.80 (1.10)		
CIQ- Total Score				
CBT	17.90 (4.45)	17.16 (5.67)	11.93 (8.26)	11.43 (4.84)
EMD	15.98 (9.32)	15.87 (6.09)	16.84 (6.13)	18.77 (1.75)
Controls	16.76 (6.32)	21.62 (3.77)*		

Note. The EMD and CBT groups each had 8 participants and the Control group had 6 participants. After being wait-listed, six control participants were assigned to the CBT and EMD groups. On the CIQ- Home subscale and Total score, higher scores indicate better reported daily functioning. On the MC Inventory-Present Ability subscale, higher scores indicate better perceived memory ability. * = $p < 0.05$ ** = $p < 0.01$.

CIQ. There was a significant pre-to-post training effect on EMD participants' daily functioning. Paired t-tests showed that following intervention the EMD group reported better functioning in their daily home activities (CIQ- Home subscale: $p < .05$), although they did not report better functioning in their daily social or productive activities (CIQ- Social and Productive subscales: $p > .05$). By 3-month follow-up, the EMD group no longer reported significantly better functioning in their daily home activities. There were no significant pre-to-post intervention effects for the CBT group. The study partners' ratings of participants' daily functioning did not differ from pre-to-post training except that the wait-list controls' study partners rated their participants' overall functioning in daily home, social, and productive activities as improved from the first to the second baseline (CIQ- Total score: $p < .05$).

MC Inventory. There were significant pre-to-post training effects on participants' perceived memory ability. Following intervention the CBT group perceived their present memory ability to be better (Present Ability Scale: $p < .01$), although they did not perceive to have better control over their memory (Potential Improvement Scale: $p > .05$; Effort Utility Scale: $p > .05$; Independence Scale: $p >.05$; AD Likelihood Scale $p > .05$; Inevitable Decline Scale: $p >.05$). By 3-month follow-up, the CBT group did not still report significantly better perceived memory ability. However, from the first to the second baseline, the control group showed higher perceived memory ability as well (Present Ability Scale: $p < .05$).

Other outcome measures. There were no significant pre-to-post intervention effects on participants' quality of life, mood, or participants' objective memory performance (HVLT-R). There were no significant pre-to-post intervention effects on participants' reported use of memory compensation strategies. However, there was a statistical trend following intervention. The CBT group reported using memory compensation strategies more frequently overall (MCQ- Total Score: $p < .07$).

Comparison ratings between participants and study partners. There were no significant differences between participants and study partners' ratings of participants' daily functioning or subjective memory appraisal at the beginning or end of the program.

Conclusion

Our pilot study examined the feasibility of two behavioral interventions to improve daily function, mood, and quality of life in individuals with amnestic MCI. Our primary goals were to explore ways to assist MCI patients in compensating for memory problems and to expand knowledge about the challenges associated with implementing this type of intervention with MCI patients. Results indicate that the EMD group reported significantly better functioning in their daily activities at home following training. However, perceived improved daily activities at home did not persist at the 3- and 6-month follow-up assessments and was not confirmed by study partners. Previous studies have suggested that collateral reports of MCI patients' abilities to perform complex activities of daily living are more reliable than patient reports (Tabert, et al., 2002), so this result should be interpreted with caution. Although study partner ratings of participant daily functioning did not increase following training, they did not decrease from baseline either. This may be important, since this stable period of functional ability reported by study partners lasted 6 months for some participants. Interestingly, there was significant improvement in study partner ratings of the wait-list control group's overall daily functioning from first to second baseline ($p < .05$). One possible explanation is that study partners of participants in the intervention groups had some expectation of improvement in daily functioning and therefore rated more harshly.

In contrast with the Tabert, et al. study (2002), we found no significant differences between participant and study partner ratings of participants' daily functioning. Our MCI participants were more aware of their memory problems and functional abilities and appraised them more realistically. Additionally, we found no significant differences between participant and study partner ratings of participants' subjective memory complaints, although participants and study partners reported different memory concerns. Participants reported the most problems remembering names, while their study partners reported they were having the most problem remembering conversations. Interventions might be most fruitful if they are individualized to target compensatory strategies for types of memory most concerning to patients' and collaterals such as, in this case, remembering names and conversations (Scherer, 2005). Additionally, these findings highlight the importance of assessing collaterals' reports of patients' cognitive decline in addition to patients' reports of memory complaints when making diagnostic decisions about MCI.

The CBT group had significantly better subjective memory appraisals and a statistical trend indicated that they used memory compensation strategies more frequently following training. Therefore, it appears that training with cognitive-behavioral therapy techniques targeting participants' subjective memory appraisals had benefits. However, perceived better subjective memory appraisals did not persist at the 3- and 6-month follow-ups and the wait-list control group reported better subjective memory appraisals from the first to second baseline. Thus, these results should be interpreted with caution. As predicted, neither group showed improvement on objective memory testing following training.

Contrary to our predictions, neither group reported improved quality of life or mood following training. There are several possible reasons for these results. First, the questionnaire we used to measure quality of life may have been too general to detect specific changes associated with the program. Second, our participants reported relatively high quality of life and mood at the onset of training, so treatment effects would be difficult to achieve. Although subjects did not report improved mood or quality of life, all participants reported that they benefited from the program by getting to know other people with similar concerns and study partners agreed that the experience was positive. Both participants and study partners believed that if the program had been shorter, this benefit would have been lost.

The inclusion of study partners was helpful in multiple ways. First, study partners learned, along with the participants, about how the brain stores memories and which memories are more fragile than others. In addition, they were helpful in reminding participants to follow-through with home exercises. For the CBT group, study partners were educated about the emotional reactions that can accompany memory problems and how negative responses can exacerbate memory failures. Furthermore, they could observe and practice role modeling of constructive responses to memory failures with their participants. For the EMD group, the study partners were critical for assisting the participants learn new skills. We learned that study partners in the home were more effective than a family member or friend living outside the home. Finally, we learned that it was just as important for study partners to be motivated to participate in the program as it was for participants.

In general, participants in the CBT group reported that the non- electronic aids were "very useful" and reported continued use of the aids daily at the end of training and at follow-up. In contrast, participants in the EMD group reported that the electronic aids were "somewhat" to "not useful" and reported "occasional" to "no" use of the electronic aids at the end of training and at follow-up. Many participants in the EMD group reported that they enjoyed the challenge of learning to use electronic aids; however, they proved too complicated and participants stopped using them after the program ended.

Even though participants reported misplacing objects as one of their frequent problems, they did not find the electronic object locators useful or beneficial. The receivers were larger than desirable and many people reported that they never knew in advance what they were going to misplace. Others did not like the requirement that they had to be in the same room as the object to hear the auditory signal. Advantages of the digital voice recorder were that it was small, lightweight, and allowed for skipping from one message to the next. However, the disadvantages were that it was too small to read the screen easily and it was confusing and difficult to operate. For example, it took three steps to erase a message. Advantages of the microcassette recorder were that it was easier to operate. However, the disadvantages were that it was larger, the buttons were not well marked, and did not skip from one message to the next. Advantages of the simple personal digital assistant (PDA) were that it was small and lightweight. Disadvantages were that it was too small to read the screen easily and it was complicated to operate.

The present study used off-the-shelf, readily available electronic devices. Recently, there has been renewed focus on designing electronic devices to be more usable by aging adults (Arning and Ziefle, 2007; Czaja and Lee, 2007; Zajicek, 2004; Ziefle and Bay, 2005). Issues of screen and button size, complexity of the interface, and the ease of learning the interface are now recognized to be important factors to the uptake of these devices by older adults. Sensory and motor limitations of both participants and study partners need to be considered when implementing an MCI intervention program. Importantly, the electronic devices selected need to have easy to read displays and feature labels, and alarms need to be adjustable for loudness required by age-associated hearing loss.

In a study of young and older adults, Arning and Ziefle (2007) found a significant association between performance using a PDA and the perceived usefulness and ease of use for older adults. This problem is likely exacerbated in individuals with MCI, who may have low expectations of their ability to use a new electronic device. One of the major challenges in training our participants to use electronic devices was that many did not use electronic items such as computers and cell phones in their daily lives, and thus preferred aids they were comfortable and confident using, like paper and pencil items. Since perceived control is potentially important to the implementation of memory strategies, it would have been ideal to pair CBT strategies with the more difficult to master electronic aids in the EMD intervention. However, a CBT component was not added to the EMD intervention because the study was exploratory in nature and we chose to equate the lengths of two different pilot interventions. Future programs should focus multiple sessions training participants how to use each electronic device through errorless learning instruction in combination with using cognitive-behavioral techniques such as cognitive restructuring to build participants' sense of confidence and skill mastery.

One limitation of this study is reliance on self-report data. Therefore, we cannot say how often participants actually used memory compensation aids or how they actually performed in their daily activities. Future studies should use performance-based measures of memory aid use and daily functioning in addition to self-report measures; for instance, electronic devices that are programmed to record when on or used. Additionally, full randomization of participants into groups was not possible. Due to varying intervals between MCI diagnosis and start of the program, participants' levels of cognitive impairment may have progressed and could be associated with limited benefits associated with the program. Furthermore, there may have been treatment effects at six months, although the results are all non-significant due most likely to the very limited sample size and statistical power at the six-month follow-up. Finally, of all the individuals who were contacted to participate in the study, we recruited only 18 couples due mainly to the time and transportation commitments and strict requirements for study partners.

Because this was a clinic-based sample of well-educated community dwelling adults with amnestic MCI, it may not be appropriate to generalize the results of this study to the broader population of adults with MCI. More mood disturbance, dependency on others, and differences in perception of memory and functional abilities between participants and study partners might be observed in other sample populations. In general, our difficulty recruiting motivated and well-educated patients with less than expected mood disturbance implies that it would be difficult to recruit MCI patients in the broader population into similar programs. In order to reach a wider range of MCI patients, future interventions could be shorter in length and not have the requirements of personal transportation to and from sessions as well as a study partner who can attend most sessions. However, the CBT portion of the intervention may actually be more effective with MCI patients who have more mood impairment, although they may have a tendency not to volunteer for research.

The outcome measures chosen may have been too global to detect specific changes in quality of life and daily functioning associated with the interventions (i.e. QLESQ, CIQ, FAQ). Due to the lack of well-established measures of daily functioning designed for this population, we used a modified functional abilities measure designed originally for head injury patients that may not have been appropriate for use with MCI patients. Thus, future studies are needed to develop and validate such measures, particularly ones designed for intervention research.

In sum, the present findings should be used as preliminary data to help expand knowledge of issues that clinicians and investigators should consider when designing and implementing an MCI group intervention program. Our participants preferred using non-electronic aids. Clearly, the development of simple electronic memory aids designed for older adults and memory impaired populations along with further development of targeted behavioral interventions for patients with MCI are needed.

Authors' Notes

Adriana M. Seelye, M.S., Diane, B. Howieson, Ph.D., Katherine V. Wild, Ph.D., Luis R. Sauceda, B.A, and Jeffrey A. Kaye, M.D. Department of Neurology, Oregon Health and

Science University. Adriana M. Seelye is now at the Department of Psychology, Washington State University. This study was supported by the Oregon Partnership for Alzheimer's Research, the Oregon Center for Aging and Technology (P30 AG024978-03), and the NIA-Layton Aging and Alzheimer's Disease Center (P30 AG08017). Correspondence concerning this chapter should be addressed to Adriana Seelye, Department of Psychology, Washington State University, Pullman, Washington 99164-4820. Electronic mail may be sent to aseelye@wsu.edu.

References

Arning, K., and Ziefle, M. (2007). Understanding age differences in PDA acceptance and performance. Including the Special Issue: education and pedagogy with learning objects and learning designs. *Computers in Human Behavior, 23*(6), 2904-2927.

Backman, L., Josephsson, S., Herlitz, A., Stigsdotter, A., and Viitanen, M. (1991). The generalizibility of training gains in dementia: Effects of an imagery-based mnemonic on face-name retention duration. *Psychology of Aging, 6*(3), 489-492.

Ball, K., Berch, D. B., Helmers, K. F., Jobe, J. B., Leveck, M. D., Marsiske, M., et al. (2002). Effects of cognitive training interventions with older adults: a randomized controlled trial. *Journal of the American Medical Association, 288*(18), 2271-2281.

Belleville, S., Gilbert, B., Fontaine, F., Gagnon, L., Menard, E., and Gauthier, S. (2006). Improvement of episodic memory in persons with mild cognitive impairment and healthy older adults: Evidence from a cognitive intervention program. *Dementia and Geriatric Cognitive Disorders, 22*(5-6), 486-499.

Bennett, D. A., Wilson, R. S., Schneider, J. A., Evans, D. A., Beckett, L. A., Aggarwal, N. T., et al. (2002). Natural History of mild cognitive impairment in older persons. *Neurology, 59*, 198-205.

Clare, L., Wilson, B. A., Carter, G., Breen, K., Gosses, A., and Hodges, J. R. (2000). Intervening with everyday memory problems in dementia of the Alzheimer type: an errorless learning approach. *Journal of Clinical and Experimental Neuropsychology, 22*, 132-146.

Czaja, S. J., and Lee, C. C. (2007). The impact of aging on access to technology. *Universal Access in the Information Society, 5(4)*, 341-349.

Dixon, R. A., De Frias, C. M., and Backman, L. (2001). Characteristics of self-reported memory compensation in older adults. *Journal of Clinical and Experimental Neuropsychology, 23*(5), 650-661.

Endicott, J., Nee, J., Harrison, W., and Blumenthal, R. (1993). Quality of Life Enjoyment and Satisfaction Questionnaire: A new measure. *Psychopharmacology Bulletin, 29*, 321-326.

Farias, S. T., Mungas, D., Reed, B. R., Harvey, D. H., Cahn-Weiner, D., and DeCarli, C. (2006). MCI is associated with deficits in everyday living. *Alzheimer's disease and Associated Disorders, 20(*4), 217-223.

Floyd, M. and Scogin, F. (1997). Effects of memory training on the subjective memory functioning and mental health of older adults: A meta-analysis. *Psychology and Aging, 12*(1), 150-161.

Greenaway, M.C., Smith, G.E., Lepore, S., Lunde, A., Hanna, S., and Boeve, B. (2006). Compensating for memory loss in mild cognitive impairment. Poster Presentation at the 10th International Conference on Alzheimer's disease and Related Disorders, Madrid, Spain.

Hart, T., Buchhofer, R., and Vaccaro, M. (2004). Portable electronic devices as memory and organizational aids after traumatic brain injury: a consumer survey study. *Journal of Head Trauma Rehabilitation, 19*(5), 351-365.

Howieson, D. B., Camicoli, R., Quinn, J., Silbert, L. C., Care, B., Moore, M. M., et al. (2003). Natural history of cognitive decline in the oldest old. *Neurology*, *60*(9), 1484-1494.

Lachman, M. E., Weaver, S. L., Bandura, M., Elliott, E., and Lewkowicz, C. J. (1992). Improving memory and control beliefs through cognitive restructuring and self-generated strategies. *Journal of Gerontology, 47*(5), 293-299.

Lachman, M. E., Weaver, S. L., and Elliot, E. (1995). Assessing memory control beliefs: the memory controllability inventory. *Aging and Cognition, 2*, 67-84.

Loewenstein, D. A., Acevedo, A., Czaja, S. J., and Dura, R. (2004). Cognitive rehabilitation of mildly impaired Alzheimer disease patients on cholinesterase inhibitors. *American Journal of Geriatric Psychiatry, 12*(4), 395-402.

Lowenstein, D. A., Barker, W. W., Harwood, D. G., Luis, C., Avecedo, A., Rodriguez, I., et al. (2000). Utility of a modified Mini-Mental State Examination with extended delayed recall in screening for mild cognitive impairment and dementia among community dwelling elders. *International Journal of Geriatric Psychiatry, 15*, 434-440.

Mimura, M., and Komatsu, S. (2007). Cognitive rehabilitation and cognitive training for mild dementia. *Psychogeriatrics*, *7*(3), 137-143.

Mohs, R. C., Ashman, T. A., Jantzen, K., Albert, M., Brandt, J., Gordon, B., et al. (1998). A study of the efficacy of a comprehensive memory enhancement program in healthy elderly persons. *Psychiatry Research, 77*(3), 183-195.

O'Neil-Pirozzi, T. M., Kendrick, H., Goldstein, R., and Glenn, M. (2004). Clinician influences on use of portable electronic memory devices in traumatic brain injury rehabilitation. *Brain Injury, 18*(2), 179-189.

Onor, M. L., Trevisiol, M., Negro, C., Alessandra, S., Saina, M., and Aguglia, E. (2007) Impact of a multimodal rehabilitative intervention on demented patients and their caregivers. *American Journal of Alzheimer's Disease and Other Dementias, 22*(4), 261-272.

Oriani, M., Moniz-Cook, E., Binetti, G., Zanieri, G., Frisoni, G .B., Geroldi, C., et al. (2003). An electronic memory aid to support prospective memory in patients in the early stages of Alzheimer's disease: A pilot study. *Aging and Mental Health, 7*(1), 22-27.

Pfeffer, R. I., Kurosaki, T. T., Harrah, C. H., Jr., Chance, J. M., and Filos, S. (1982). Measurement of functional activities in older adults in the community. *Journal of Gerontology, 37*(3), 323-329.

Rapp, S. R., Brenes, G., and Marsh, A. P. (2002). Memory enhancement training for older adults with mild cognitive impairment: A preliminary study. *Aging and Mental Health, 6*(1), 5-11.

Scherer, M. J. (2005). Assessing the benefits of using assistive technologies and other supports for thinking, remembering, and learning. *Disability and Rehabilitation, 27*(13), 731-739.

Schmitter-Edgecombe, M., Howard, J. T., Pavawalla, S., Howell, L. and Rueda, A. (in press). Multi-dyad Memory Notebook Intervention for Very Mild Dementia: A Pilot Study. *American Journal of Alzheimer's Disease and Other Dementias.*

Shapiro, A. M., Benedict, R. H., Schretlen, D., and Brandt, J. (1999). Construct and concurrent validity of the Hopkins Verbal Learning Test-revised. *Clinical Neuropsychology, 13*(3), 348-358.

Singer, T., Lindenberger, U., and Baltes, P. B. (2003). Plasticity of memory for new learning in very old age: A story of major loss? *Psychology and Aging, 18*(2), 306-317.

Sitzer, D. I., Twamley, E. W., and Jeste, D. V. (2006). Cognitive training in Alzheimer's disease: a meta-analysis of the literature. *Acta Psychiatrica Scandinavica, 114*, 75–90.

Sohlberg, M. M., Ehlhardt, L., and Kennedy, M. (2005). Instructional techniques in cognitive rehabilitation: A preliminary report. *Seminars in Speech and Language, 26*(4), 268-279.

Tabert, M. H., Albert, S. M., Borvkhova-Milov, L., Camacho, Y., Pelton, G., Liu, X., et al. (2002). Functional deficits in individuals with mild cognitive impairment: prediction of Alzheimer's disease. *American Academy of Neurology, 58*(5), 758-764.

Talassi, E., Guerreschi, M., Feriani, M., Fedi, V., Bianchetti, A., and Trabucchi, M. (2007).
Effectiveness of a cognitive rehabilitation program in mild dementia (MD) and mild cognitive impairment (MCI): A case control study. *Archives of Gerontology and Geriatrics, 44*(S1), 391-399.

van den Broek, M. D., Downes, J., Johnson, Z., Dayus, B., and Hilton, N. (2000). Evaluation of an electronic memory aid in the neuropsychological rehabilitation of prospective memory deficits. *Brain Injury, 14*(5), 455-462.

Wadley, V. G., Crowe, M., Marsiske, M., Cook, S. E., Unverzagt, F. W., Rosenberg, A. L., et al. (2007). Changes in everyday function in individuals with psychometrically defined mild cognitive impairment in the Advanced Cognitive Training for Independent and Vital Elderly Study. *Journal of the American Geriatrics Society, 55*(8), 1192-1198.

Willer, B., Rosenthal, M., Kreutzer, J. S., Gordon, W., and Rempel, R. (1993). Assessment of community integration following rehabilitation for traumatic brain injury. *Journal of Head Trauma Rehabilitation, 8*, 75-87.

Wilson, B. A., Baddeley, A., Evans, J., and Shiel, A. (1994). Errorless learning in the rehabilitation of memory impaired people. *Neuropsychological Rehabilitation , 4,* 307-326.

Winblad, B., Palmer, K., Kivipelto, M., Jelic, V., Fratiglioni, L., Wahlund, L.-O., et al. (2004). Mild cognitive impairment—beyond controversies, towards a consensus: Report of the International Working Group on Mild Cognitive Impairment. *Journal of Internal Medicine, 256*(3), 240-246.

Yesavage, J. A. (1988). Geriatric Depression Scale. *Psychopharmacology Bulletin, 24*(4), 709-711.

Zajicek, M. (2004). Successful and available: Interface design exemplars for older users. *Interacting with Computers Universal Usability Revised, 16*(3), 411-430.

Zelinski, E. M., Gilewski, M. J., and Anthony-Bergstone, C. R. (1990). Memory Functioning Questionnaire: Concurrent validity with memory performance and self-reported memory failures. *Psychology and Aging, 5*, 388-399.

Ziefle, M., and Bay, S. (2005). How older adults meet complexity: Aging effects on the usability of different mobile phones. *Behaviour and Information Technology, 24*(5), 375-389.

In: New Directions in Aging Research
Editor: Ruby R. Brougham, pp. 75-90
ISBN 978-1-60741-976-1
© 2009 Nova Science Publishers, Inc.

Chapter 5

Multidimensional Pain Assessment in Geriatric Oncology: An Innovative Approach

Chih-Hung Chang *

Northwestern University, Feinberg School of Medicine, Chicago, Illinois, USA

Abstract

Pain is a complex multidimensional and subjective experience. It is the most common complaint of patients seeking medical treatment and a frequent symptom of older adults. Pain in geriatric oncology (gero-oncology) is a pressing issue given the demographic trends pointing to an increasing population of older cancer patients, for whom pain will be a significant consequence. Although a critical mass of pain assessment tools now exist, there routine use in clinical practice has not reached the desired levels due to logistical constraints. Accurate multidimensional pain assessment in gero-oncology is challenging, but necessary, first step to optimize personalized pain treatment and management. The Clinical Infometrics approach that integrates modern test theory and advanced technology offers a fruitful venue for resolving many measurement issues. Well-designed computerized methodologies can potentially streamline the process of patient assessment and increase the accessibility of data to the interdisciplinary team of healthcare professionals (including physicians, nurses, and social workers). This chapter summarizes the challenges of pain assessment in gero-oncology patients specifically and discusses plausible solutions to overcome these challenges using innovative methodologies and technologies.

* Address correspondence to: Chih-Hung Chang, Ph.D., Buehler Center on Aging, Health and Society, Feinberg School of Medicine, Northwestern University. 750 N. Lake Shore Dr., Suite 601, Chicago, IL 60611. Phone: (312) 503-4354; Fax: (312) 503-5868; E-mail: chchang@northwestern.edu

Introduction

Pain is the most common complaint of patients seeking medical treatment, and it is a frequent symptom of older adults. Pain is a multidimensional and subjective experience. It is a frequent symptom among older adults and often under-treated (Aguglia, 2000; DeWaters, Popovich, and Faut-Callahan, 2003; Frampton, 2003; Nikolaus and Zeyfang, 2004; Sheehan and Forman, 1997; Stiefel and Stagno, 2004; Yun, et al., 2003). Aging may lead to decreased pain tolerance in elders, and pain prevalence for those older than age 60 is estimated to be doubled that of people under age 60. The high prevalence of pain in older adults makes it a pressing public health issue, yet few studies of pain relief focus on older adults (Gloth, 2000; Portenoy, Ugarte, Fuller, and Haas, 2004). Pain may have impacts for elders beyond the symptom of pain itself, as it correlates with lower self-rated health, depression, and fatigue, anxiety and distress (Crook, Rideout, and Browne, 1984; Fox, Raina, and Jadad, 1999; Mantyselka, Turunen, Ahonen, and Kumpusalo, 2003). Despite these numerous negative health effects, patients 85 years or older were less likely to receive analgesics compared with younger patients (Ohayon and Schatzberg, 2003).

Pain in Geriatric Oncology (Gero-Oncology)

Cancer is an excellent model for understanding how pain assessment, treatment, and management related to chronic, life-threatening illness treatment preference over time, particularly in this elderly population. Geriatric oncology (gero-oncology) has become an important sub-discipline in medicine due to the rapidly growing population of elderly patients, many of whom have cancer. Pain will be significant consequence for the gero-oncology patients. As the elderly population is becoming more diverse, more attention will need to be paid to the heterogeneous and complex factors that influence the experience of multidimensional pain. Pain is the most common complaint of advanced cancer patients, and its effective management in the older cancer patients requires on-going assessment and a multi-modal treatment approach that accommodates age-related processes. Incomplete pain assessment has been described as a significant barrier to cancer pain management (Spiegel, Sands, and Koopman, 1994).

Accurate pain assessment in gero-oncology is challenging but a necessary first step in order to optimize individual pain treatment and management. Initial assessment, prompt treatment, and regular reassessment of pain are essential so that gero-oncology patients can receive a more tailored care to improve their quality of life. A plethora of pain assessment tools exist, but only a few are for the assessment of gero-oncology pain and its specific domains. Gaps also exist in the areas of practical, comprehensive, condition-specific, and culturally-sensitive data acquisition methods which capture clinically-meaningful data about patient pain. Also needed is a psychometrically robust, precise indicator of patient-rated pain which is interpretable by clinicians and useful for research analyses. Using integrated methodologies and technologies, broad sources of data on gero-oncology pain in all its dimensions can be effectively collected, processed and interpreted to improve pain assessment, treatment, and management.

An Innovative Approach to Rapid and Reliable Pain Assessment

If information of pain assessment is to be used effectively in pain treatment and management, it must be psychometrically sound, clinically relevant, and readily available. Several sophisticated statistical methodologies can be applied in pain measurement and evaluation. The use of IRT models (Andrich, 1988; Hambleton and Swaminathan, 1985; Hambleton, Swaminathan, and Rogers, 1991) and IRT-based computer adaptive testing (CAT) (Wainer, et al., 1990; Weiss, 1985; Weiss and Kingsbury, 1984) in health outcomes assessment has grown considerably, due to a developing consensus that IRT provides more adaptable and effective methods of measurement and scoring (McHorney, 1997, 1998, 1999). Advanced computer technologies are crucial for developing an effective program with capacity for off-site use that is especially well-suited to the elderly and other groups that lack access to health care resources. The approach to integrate both well-developed methodologies and advanced technologies can lessen the complexity of pain assessment and help reduce the failures in gero-oncology pain management.

Frameworks of Multidimensional Pain

While pain is generally accepted as a multidimensional construct, few assessment tools have fully addressed this multidimensionality. In constructing a comprehensive assessment tool for gero-oncology pain, it is essential to have a starting point that is grounded in frameworks that have successfully integrated a multidimensional or multi-domain understanding of human suffering and illness. Below we review the biopsychosocial and palliative care models of medicine that will serve as the theoretical basis for the identification of domains of importance.

Biopsychosocial Model of Medicine

The biomedical model of health has been extraordinarily fruitful, but it has not explained the existence of socio-demographic predictors of health. The biopsychosocial (BPS) model of medicine, first introduced by Engel, integrates other domains (the psychological and social, in addition to the biological) that present a more complete picture of the patient (Engel, 1977). The variant Interactive Biopsychosocial Model (IBM) takes a more systems-based approach that may be more appropriate to clinical settings (Lindau, Laumann, Levinson, and Waite, 2003). The BPS approach has been applied to a variety of pain conditions, such as chronic upper limb, chest, low back, multiple sclerosis, rheumatoid arthritis, and cancer (Covic, Adamson, Spencer, and Howe, 2003; Henderson, Kidd, Pearson, and White, 2005; Kerns, Kassirer, and Otis, 2002; Sutton, Porter, and Keefe, 2002; Thurston, Keefe, Bradley, Rama Krishnan, and Caldwell, 2001; Truchon, 2001). The BPS model has been applied to investigations of the psychological and social variables in cancer pain (Keefe, et al., 2003; Zimmerman, Story, Gaston-Johansson, and Rowles, 1996). Some of these non-biological variables have been shown to be significant predictors of pain, albeit weaker than biomedical variables (Syrjala and Chapko, 1995). However, while the BPS model of pain has influenced medical research, it has not fully taken root in medical practice. One of the ways to bridge this gap between research and practice is to integrate the principles of the BPS model into health care provision routines, beginning with assessment.

Palliative Care Model of Medicine

Palliative care has spread dramatically due to its ability to meet the needs of patients and families dealing with cancer and end-of-life issues (Saunders, 1959). Based first upon consensus statements, then on empirical research grounded in the experience of patients and families, and most recently on standards of care, essentially similar depictions of the conceptual frameworks have emerged for palliative care (Emanuel, Alpert, Baldwin, and Emanuel, 2000; Lynn, 1997; National Institutes of Health, 2002; Singer, Martin, and Kelner, 1999; Steinhauser, et al., 2000). Despite some differences, these models propose four domains that are relevant to the patient experience: physical, mental, social, and existential. Palliative care has already been helpful in improving measures for symptom control (Bruera, Kuehn, Miller, Selmser, and Macmillan, 1991; Chang, Hwang, and Feuerman, 2000; Chang, Hwang, Feuerman, Kasimis, and Thaler, 2000). In addition, the importance of existential variables in pain have been documented (Portenoy, et al., 1994). The social and emotional dimensions of illness and its burdens are also now receiving attention (Covinsky, et al., 1999; Strang, 1998). Palliative care and medicine in general would benefit from refined items and measures for the measurement and subsequent management of cancer pain, starting with a geriatric population and eventually expanding to other subpopulations.

Pain Assessment

Pain Is Multidimensional and Subjective

Pain has been defined by the International Association for the Study on Pain Subcommittee on Taxonomy as "an unpleasant sensory and emotional experience associated with actual or potential tissue damage or described in terms of such damage (International Association for the Study of Pain, 1986)." Pain is a multidimensional experience with many contributing and interacting biological mechanisms. However, pain is also a subjective experience. Several disciplines have attempted to reveal the multiple underlying dimensions of the experience of pain in order to contribute to an overarching biopsychosocial model (Turk and Monarch, 2002). Currently popular pain assessment tools used in clinical evaluations can be improved by integration of research on self-report, memory processes and pain, and particularly research on the "language of pain" (Hinnant, 2002). Expressions concerning the intensity and duration of pain are largely metaphorical, and culturally variable (Moore and Dworkin, 1988; Schott, 2004), as Spanish adaptations of the McGill Pain Questionnaire make evident (Escalante, Lichtenstein, Lawrence, Roberson, and Hazuda,

1996; Lazaro, et al., 2001). However, even non-linguistic indicators show ethnic and racial differences as has been shown for research on the Visual Analog Scale with African-Americans and whites (Cassisi, et al., 2004). Cultural variables have also been shown to define the way pain is perceived and treated among cancer patients. Differences have been noted in pain perception of elderly Caucasians and African Americans experiencing short-term pain and Hispanic patients experiencing cancer-related pain.

Comprehensive Pain Assessment

Comprehensive assessment of cancer-related pain is essential to finding the best treatment options. Three major sources of information about pain exist: verbal report, behavioral measures, and physiological measures. Although its multidimensional nature is well recognized, pain is often assessed as a unitary dimension. The most common unidimensional measures assess the physical domain and pain intensity scales that use visual analogue or numerical ratings. More complex measures assess multiple dimensions of pain and many measures exist that assess different dimensions. For instance, the Multidimensional Pain Inventory purports to measure the physical, psychological, and social domains (Kerns, Turk, and Rudy, 1985); however, several of the items may not be relevant to an older cancer population, and there are no items that address the spiritual domain, which the palliative care model suggests may be important in cancer pain.

Table 1. Samples of Existing Pain Measures

Measure	Type of Pain	Scale	No. of Items	Respondent (minutes)
Visual Analogue Pain Rating Scale	General pain	Ratio	1	Self (0.5)
McGill Pain Questionnaire	General pain	Ordinal, Interval	20	Self (15-20)
Brief Pain Inventory	Cancer pain	Ordinal	20	Self (10-15)
Medical Outcomes Study Pain Measures	General pain	Ordinal	12	Self
Illness Behavior Questionnaire	Maladaptive responses to pain	Ordinal	52	Self
Pain and Distress Scale	Mood/Behavior changes due to pain	Ordinal	20	Self
Pain Perception Profile	General pain	Ratio	37	Expert
Geriatric Pain Measure	Geriatric pain	Dichotomous, Interval	24	Self (< 5)
West Haven-Yale Multidimensional Pain Inventory	Chronic pain	Ordinal	52	Self
Pain Disability Index	Chronic pain/disability	Ordinal	7	Self
Dartmouth Pain Questionnaire	General pain	Ordinal, Interval	5	Self (5-20)
Pain Patient Profile	General pain	Ordinal	44	Self (15)
Abbey Pain Scale	Geriatric pain	Ordinal	6	Expert (5)

While the many pain assessment tools may confuse the end-users with a variety of questions, rating scales (response categories), and summary scores, this diversity is valuable as it provides the researchers or clinicians with choices based upon specific disease site characteristics or pain domains of interest. However, one practical problem of pain assessment is that pain measures have diverse scaling properties. These questionnaires vary in a number of ways including the scale length, number of response categories, reference periods, and target populations (see Table 1 for example).

A resource is needed that pools items from high quality existing questionnaires. This would allow the creation of brief questionnaires using the most informative questions or individually tailored questionnaires with only the minimal number of adaptively derived questions. Item response theory (IRT) modeling (described later) provides a vehicle for both needs by supplying the methods for creating item banks. Creating a viable pain item bank would require reconciliation of these various instruments, subjecting them to psychometric analysis so that items could be drawn in real time for specific purposes or patient populations.

Challenges in Pain Assessment in Geriatrics

Despite the benefits of patient-reported pain information, they are not routinely collected and used in clinical practice. Well-designed computerized methodologies can potentially streamline the process of patient assessment and increase the accessibility of data to the interdisciplinary team of healthcare professionals (including physicians, nurses, and social workers). We discuss three primary challenges among others in comprehensive geriatric pain assessment below.

Lack of Adequate Computerized Delivery Platforms

Most barriers to successful pain information gathering can be attributed to the use of the paper-and-pencil data collection method, which is labor-intensive for administration, data processing and analysis. Computerized pain assessment, if designed properly, offers some promises. For instance, a portable computing device such as a Tablet PC with voice recognition would be a good alternative for patients without sufficient physical strength or energy to answer pain questions. These scenarios highlight the importance of supporting multiple delivery platforms in order to elicit information about the pain experience from patients with diverse demographics (e.g., level of education or health literacy and cultural background) and clinical characteristics (e.g., stage of illness and physical condition).

Respondent Burden

Clinical research oriented questionnaires are often lengthy (more than 20 items) and usually overburden patients. The respondent burden may lead to future disinterest in taking pain assessments and can cause resource contention issues when administered at clinics (e.g., a patient may need to stay in the exam room longer to complete the assessment). The problem of patient overburden is exacerbated when multiple domains in a battery of questionnaires need to be measured in one assessment session. Using traditional fixed-length questionnaires, it becomes unrealistic to ask elderly patients to fill out multiple questionnaires on a consistent basis, especially for the elderly.

Lack of Consolidated, Comprehensive Clinically Relevant Pain Items

Clinicians want clinically relevant questions that can be aggregated and made available during the same medical encounter. Different types of pain manifest differently and therefore likely need particular sets of questions for specific areas of concern. A consolidated pain item bank covering all the relevant domains (e.g. location, frequency, intensity, and impact) is an effective and economical approach that benefits both patients and physicians. A well-designed pain item bank can then be fine-tuned to suit the needs of different disease sites, instead of being overly generic, although these site-specific item banks could share certain items that are of common concern.

Innovative Methodologies and Technologies

Although cancer pain is multidimensional and subjective, it should be assessed with sufficient rigor to prompt optimal treatment. Modern psychometric theory (i.e., IRT), routinely applied in educational testing psychological assessment, offers a fruitful venue for examining the psychometric properties of instruments purported to assess the multidimensional pain experience. IRT has gained its popularity and acceptance in health assessment because it provides more adaptable and effective methods of scale construction, analysis, and scoring which complement those derived from classical test theory (Chang and Reeve, 2005). Pain assessment and management can also be augmented with advanced technologies (e.g., Personal Digital Assistant, SmartPhone, iPhone) for the assessment of pain in diverse settings including homes, clinical practice and care settings (assisted living, skilled care, and nursing homes) to allow for personalized pain management.

Item Response Theory (IRT)

IRT is a family of mathematical models used to determine the characteristics (e.g., "difficulty" or "severity") of test items or survey questions and to estimate the level of latent traits (e.g., "ability" or "pain") of persons on the same underlying construct being measured. The three most popular unidimensional IRT models are the one-, two-, and three-parameter logistic (PL) models (see Table 2), so named because of the number of item parameters each incorporates (Hambleton and Swaminathan, 1985). Unidimensional dichotomous models are appropriate for binary response (e.g., yes/no) or dichotomously-scored (e.g., right/wrong) items.

Table 2. Unidimensional Dichotomous Response Models

Models	Mathematical Forms	Item Parameter
One-Parameter Logistic	$P_i(\theta) = \frac{1}{1+e^{-D(\theta-b_i)}}$	Difficulty (b)
Two-Parameter Logistic	$P_i(\theta) = \frac{1}{1+e^{-Da_i(\theta-b_i)}}$	Difficulty (b), Discrimination (a)
Three-Parameter Logistic	$P_i(\theta) = c_i + (1-c_i)\frac{1}{1+e^{-Da_i(\theta-b_i)}}$	Difficulty (b), Discrimination (a), Guessing (c)

Table 3. Examples of Pain Domains and Items

Domain	Items
Physical / Biological	Intensity, Location, Quality, Duration, others
Social	Items from Multidimensional Pain Inventory, others
Psychological	Items from Pain and Distress Scale, others
Spiritual	Newly written items
New Domain #1: Behavior	Items from Illness Behavior Questionnaire, others
New Domain #2: Unknown	Newly written items

Polytomous IRT models for multi-category response (e.g., strongly disagree, disagree, agree, strongly agree) are modeled to represent the nonlinear relationship between a person trait level and the probability of responding in a particular response category, including: Bock's nominal response model; Samejima's graded response model; Andrich's rating scale model; Masters' partial credit model; and Muraki's generalized partial credit model (Andrich, 1978a, 1978b, 1978c; Bock, 1972; Masters, 1982; Muraki, 1992; Samejima, 1969, 1972). Multidimensional IRT models have also been developed to model the relationships in a matrix of responses to a set of test items.

Scale Construction

IRT provides a methodology to assess the location of an item on the latent trait continuum (i.e., item threshold parameter) and the extent to which an item is related to the underlying construct being measured (i.e., item slope or discrimination parameter). The item parameters help test developers to decide whether to remove or retain an item. In addition, when data do not fit the model requirement, ill-performed items are identifiable from the fit statistics. The fit statistics provide evidence regarding the validity of the IRT models and indices of the coherence of items to a single construct. If the fit is unacceptable, the data can be improved by eliminating the items that show a poor fit.

Differential Item Functioning (DIF)

In order to make meaningful cross-group comparisons, it is essential to use unbiased measurement tools that can detect real differences between groups. Items exhibiting DIF across groups are a serious threat to the validity of an instrument and may reduce the validity of between-group comparisons, because scores may be indicative of attributes other than those the scale is intended to measure (Thissen, Steinberg, and Wainer, 1988). An item is said to exhibit DIF, or the presence of statistical item bias, if two respondents with equal level of the trait being measured do not have the same probability of endorsing each response category of the same item when they take in a test. IRT-based DIF analysis is one way to detect whether particular items function differently among respondents in identifiable groups (e.g., male vs. female).

Instrument Linking and Equating

The primary purpose of linking or equating items from different measures is to make scores comparable (i.e., converting scores obtained from one measure to another). Analogous to converting the degrees on a thermometer from Centigrade to Fahrenheit, the purpose of linking or equating scores from different measures is to generate comparable scores from one tool to another. In other words, two responders taking different assessments (i.e., sets of questions) scaled on the same metric can have comparable scores. IRT co-calibrated items can be linked together on a common metric to allow for the creation of new measures with different sets of items from the combined item pool depending on the purpose of assessment and target population.

Item Bank

An item bank, more than just a collection or pool of items, is comprised of carefully IRT-calibrated items that define and quantify a common theme or trait. It is a prerequisite for successful adaptive testing (described below). A bank is as good as its coverage of the entire continuum of the latent trait being measured. A well constructed pain item bank (i.e., items are hierarchically arrayed) can provide a basis for selecting the best possible set of questions for any particular patient.

It is also possible to compare the scores of patients who complete different sets of questions from the same bank. Not only does this allow for tailored, "adaptive," testing, it also allows one to compare pain scores of patients across studies which have used different sets of items or scales. Finally, an item bank with wide ranging items also enables researchers or clinicians to select items to construct a customized short form depending on the target population of interest and the purpose of the assessment.

Computerized Adaptive Testing (CAT)

CAT integrates IRT methods and computer technologies to administer an assessment tool by adaptively selecting items on the basis of a patient's response to previously administered items (Wainer, et al., 2000; Weiss, 1982, 1985; Weiss and Kingsbury, 1984). CAT utilizes an iterative algorithm consisting of administering an item, estimating a person's latent trait level, and selecting the next best or informative item from an item bank to administer until some pre-determined stopping rule (e.g., minimal standard error, content coverage, or maximum scale length) is met. Each person only answers a subset of targeted items to obtain an accurate estimate of a person's score if s/he had answered all items. CAT has several advantages over conventional paper-and-pencil tests because it: 1) requires fewer questions to arrive at an accurate estimate (without loss of precision); 2) allows immediate feedback on person's health status; 3) allows users to communicate with one another on a common metric; 4) tailors item and test difficulty dynamically to the trait level of the individual; 5) eliminates the problem of excessive floor or ceiling effects; and 6) automates question administration, data recording, and scoring; therefore, human clerical errors are eliminated.

Multidimensional Adaptive Pain Assessment in Gero-Oncology

Comprehensive Pain Item Bank

Creating a comprehensive pain item bank for successful CAT implementation in gero-oncology pain is a multi-step process and requires attention to several details. It is a very time-consuming task, similar to that of creating static measures, with the additional steps for IRT modeling. It is crucial to define what is intended to measure and include sufficient number of item to cover the continuum of that construct in the item bank. The first task is to identify and refine the key domains of gero-oncology pain, using existing theoretical frameworks in biopsychosocial medicine and palliative care as a guide. The target pain measurement domains should include pain-specific domains (severity, intensity, and sources of pain) and general domains impacted by pain (physical, mental, social, and spiritual). Some of these domains are generic while others are specific to a particular type of cancer.

Second, one can systematically compile items pertinent to these multidimensional domains from existing questionnaires, writing new items for un-covered domains (see Table 3) for example.

For instance, items for the Psychological domain could be found in the Pain and Distress Scale while items for a potential new Behavior domain could be derived from the Illness Behavior Questionnaire. Domain Items extracted from these instruments will then be organized and reviewed. This resulting list of items needs to be further reviewed for clarity and redundancy.

Unidimensionality

IRT analysis requires that the item within the same scale can reasonably be considered to be reflective of one underlying dimension (sufficient unidimensionality). Therefore, a series of IRT-based analyses needs to be conducted to assess evidence for a definable underlying factor structure represented by the items for each of the scales. If a "dominant" component or factor is present, the assumption of unidimensionality can be supported.

Item and Scale Information

IRT, through the use of the logistic function, not only permits the estimation of the item and person parameters but also permits consideration of how precisely each of the parameters is estimated. A measure generally known as the information function characterizes the precision of measurement (i.e., reliability) for measuring persons at different levels of the underlying latent construct, with higher information denoting more precision. That is, a high level of information at a particular trait level can be more precisely estimated than a trait level for which the level of information is relatively low. Items with low information or items that provide redundant information (i.e., information curve overlap) may be considered for removal from the scale to create a shortened version of the instrument.

Detecting Differential Item Functioning (DIF)

Establishing item parameter invariance across different groups of gero-oncology patients is essential in building an unbiased set of items. That is, the psychometric properties of items (e.g., item discrimination and location parameters) do not change as a function of the sample. Although it is not unusual to find a certain number of items whose parameter estimates are substantially different from one group to another, studies of DIF are useful for identifying items that are problematic and require further investigation. A given item, after controlling for group differences, can exhibit DIF with respect to the slope parameter, indicating that the relationship between the item and the underlying construct is stronger in one group than in another (non-uniform DIF). DIF can also be manifested with respect to location parameters, demonstrating that the difficulty of the item varies as a function of group membership (uniform DIF). DIF analysis would allow us to determine the extent to which the items can be applied to different groups of cancer patients without compromising their psychometric properties.

Treatment of DIF Items

Items that show DIF should generally be removed from the scale, or at least not scored, if comparable scores are to be reported for all groups of respondents. However, one should first examine the magnitude and significance level of DIF, identify the potential causes of DIF, and explore the influence of background characteristics on differences in item functioning. This process will provide aid in interpreting the underlying group differences in responding to these particular items. In the longer term, the presence of DIF points to the need for further research to understand its causes using qualitative analysis technologies such as cognitive debriefing, and could ultimately lead to the development of revised questions (e.g., alternative question wordings) potentially less affected by DIF. In this way, improved cancer pain measures and deeper understanding of group differences in item responses can both be achieved.

Development of the Gero-Oncology Pain CAT

To make CAT of geriatric cancer pain a reality in clinical settings requires execution of a variety of tasks. The items included in the bank should span the full range of pain levels in this population and all item parameters must be calibrated to a common metric, as described earlier. The CAT program needs to be designed according to testing algorithms to administer pain items that cover multidimensional aspects related to cancer pain.

CATs must be delivered to each respondent on an item-by-item basis (one item at a time), with IRT calculations occurring between each item to select the next item to be administered. At the same time, good testing practice requires that test administration be standardized so that each examinee has a comparable experience (e.g., standardized screen layout).

Many of the pain scales are domain-specific and multi-indicatorial so that different types of pain outcomes can be measured on a single patient, resulting in a "profile" of indicator scores for the patient. Branching (or hierarchical) capacity can be built into the database design and CAT to deal with different types of chronic conditions, different types of quality of life domains (physical, mental, social, spiritual) or sub-domains (pain, fatigue, etc.).

Conclusion

This chapter discusses the challenges, opportunities and solutions in gero-oncology pain assessment. Quality pain assessment in gero-oncology is challenging but a necessary first step to optimize in this project will make use of well-developed methods and innovative technologies to improve assessment, the first and crucial element of improving the quality of pain management. It is essential to develop an item bank for gero-oncology pain that is rooted in the various domains of the patient experience and thus addresses the multidimensional experience of suffering. It is methodological possible to design and implement a computerized adaptive testing platform for the efficient and accurate assessment of gero-oncology pain. Ultimately, the *Pain CAT* is intended to be a multipurpose assessment program, which also has the capability to store pain items, administer fixed-length and adaptive tests, and generate reports in addition to its dynamic feature. Although we focus the condition of pain and the population of gero-oncology patients, the methods employed and discussed can be applicable to other subpopulations, including other ages, linguistic and cultural groups, and conditions.

References

Aguglia, E. (2000). Reboxetine in the maintenance therapy of depressive disorder in the elderly: a long-term open study. *International Journal of Geriatric Psychiatry, 15*(9), 784-793.

Andrich, D. (1978a). Application of a psychometric rating model to ordered categories which are scored with successive integers. *Applied Psychological Measurement, 2*(4), 581-594.

Andrich, D. (1978b). A rating formulation for ordered response categories. *Psychometrika, 43*(4), 561-573.

Andrich, D. (1978c). Scaling attitude items constructed and scored in the Likert tradition. *Educational and Psychological Measurement, 38*(3), 665-680.

Andrich, D. (1988). *Rasch models for measurement.* Newbury Park, CA: Sage Publications.

Bock, R. D. (1972). Estimating item parameters and latent ability when responses are scored in two or more nominal categories. *Psychometrika, 37*(1), 29-51.

Bruera, E., Kuehn, N., Miller, M. J., Selmser, P., and Macmillan, K. (1991). The Edmonton Symptom Assessment System (ESAS): a simple method for the assessment of palliative care patients. *Journal of Palliative Care, 7*(2), 6-9.

Cassisi, J. E., Umeda, M., Deisinger, J. A., Sheffer, C., Lofland, K. R., and Jackson, C. (2004). Patterns of pain descriptor usage in African Americans and European Americans with chronic pain. *Cultural Diversity and Ethnic Minority Psychology, 10*(1), 81-89.

Chang, C.-H., and Reeve, B. B. (2005). Item response theory and its applications to patient-reported outcomes measurement. *Evaluation and the Health Professions, 28*(3), 1-19.

Chang, V. T., Hwang, S. S., and Feuerman, M. (2000). Validation of the Edmonton Symptom Assessment Scale. *Cancer, 88*(9), 2164-2171.

Chang, V. T., Hwang, S. S., Feuerman, M., Kasimis, B. S., and Thaler, H. T. (2000). The Memorial Symptom Assessment Scale Short Form (MSAS-SF): Validity and reliability. *Cancer, 89*(5), 1162-1171.

Covic, T., Adamson, B., Spencer, D., and Howe, G. (2003). A biopsychosocial model of pain and depression in rheumatoid arthritis: a 12-month longitudinal study. *Rheumatology (Oxford), 42*(11), 1287-1294.

Covinsky, K. E., Wu, A. W., Landefeld, C. S., Connors, A. F., Jr., Phillips, R. S., Tsevat, J., et al. (1999). Health status versus quality of life in older patients: does the distinction matter? *American Journal of Medicine, 106*(4), 435-440.

Crook, J., Rideout, E., and Browne, G. (1984). The prevalence of pain complaints in a general population. *Pain, 18*(3), 299-314.

DeWaters, T., Popovich, J., and Faut-Callahan, M. (2003). An evaluation of clinical tools to measure pain in older people with cognitive impairment. *British Journal of Community Nursing, 8*(5), 226-234.

Emanuel, L. L., Alpert, H. R., Baldwin, A. H., and Emanuel, E. J. (2000). What terminally ill patients care about: toward a validated construct of patients' perspectives. *Journal of Palliative Medicine, 3*(4), 419-431.

Engel, G. L. (1977). The need for a new medical model: a challenge for biomedicine. *Science, 196*(4286), 129-136.

Escalante, A., Lichtenstein, M. J., Lawrence, V. A., Roberson, M., and Hazuda, H. P. (1996). Where does it hurt? Stability of recordings of pain location using the McGill Pain Map. *Journal of Rheumatology, 23*(10), 1788-1793.

Fox, P. L., Raina, P., and Jadad, A. R. (1999). Prevalence and treatment of pain in older adults in nursing homes and other long-term care institutions: a systematic review. *Canadian Medical Association Journal, 160*(3), 329-333.

Frampton, M. (2003). Experience assessment and management of pain in people with dementia. *Age Ageing, 32*(3), 248-251.

Gloth, F. M., 3rd. (2000). Geriatric pain. Factors that limit pain relief and increase complications. *Geriatrics, 55*(10), 46-48, 51-44.

Hambleton, R. K., and Swaminathan, H. (1985). *Item response theory : principles and applications*. Norwell, MA: Kluwer-Nijhoff Publishing.

Hambleton, R. K., Swaminathan, H., and Rogers, H. J. (1991). *Fundamentals of item response theory*. Newbury Park, CA: Sage Press.

Henderson, M., Kidd, B. L., Pearson, R. M., and White, P. D. (2005). Chronic upper limb pain: an exploration of the biopsychosocial model. *Journal of Rheumatology, 32*(1), 118-122.

Hinnant, D. W. (2002). Psychological evaluation and assessment of pain. In C. D. Tollison, J. R. Satterthwaite and J. W. Tollison (Eds.), *Practical pain management* (3rd ed., pp. 67-82). Philadelphia, Pa.: Lippincott Williams and Wilkins.

International Association for the Study of Pain. (1986). Classification of chronic pain. Descriptions of chronic pain syndromes and definitions of pain terms *Pain, 3 Suppl*, S1-226.

Keefe, F. J., Lipkus, I., Lefebvre, J. C., Hurwitz, H., Clipp, E., Smith, J., et al. (2003). The social context of gastrointestinal cancer pain: a preliminary study examining the relation of patient pain catastrophizing to patient perceptions of social support and caregiver stress and negative responses. *Pain, 103*(1-2), 151-156.

Kerns, R. D., Kassirer, M., and Otis, J. (2002). Pain in multiple sclerosis: a biopsychosocial perspective. *Journal of Rehabilitation Research and Development, 39*(2), 225-232.

Kerns, R. D., Turk, D. C., and Rudy, T. E. (1985). The West Haven-Yale Multidimensional Pain Inventory (WHYMPI). *Pain, 23*(4), 345-356.

Lazaro, C., Caseras, X., Whizar-Lugo, V. M., Wenk, R., Baldioceda, F., Bernal, R., et al. (2001). Psychometric properties of a Spanish version of the McGill Pain Questionnaire in several Spanish-speaking countries. *Clinical Journal of Pain, 17*(4), 365-374.

Lindau, S. T., Laumann, E. O., Levinson, W., and Waite, L. J. (2003). Synthesis of scientific disciplines in pursuit of health: the Interactive Biopsychosocial Model. *Perspectives in Biology and Medicine, 46*(3 Suppl), S74-86.

Lynn, J. (1997). Measuring quality of care at the end of life: a statement of principles.[see comment]. *Journal of the American Geriatrics Society, 45*(4), 526-527.

Mantyselka, P. T., Turunen, J. H., Ahonen, R. S., and Kumpusalo, E. A. (2003). Chronic pain and poor self-rated health. *Journal of the American Medical Association, 290*(18), 2435-2442.

Masters, G. N. (1982). A Rasch model for partial credit scoring. *Psychometrika, 47*(2), 149-174.

McHorney, C. A. (1997). Generic health measurement: past accomplishments and a measurement paradigm for the 21st century. *Annals of Internal Medicine, 127*(8 Pt 2), 743-750.

McHorney, C. A. (1998). Methodological inquiries in health status assessment. *Medical Care, 36*(4), 445-448.

McHorney, C. A. (1999). Health status assessment methods for adults: past accomplishments and future challenges. *Annual Review of Public Health, 20*, 309-335.

Moore, R. A., and Dworkin, S. F. (1988). Ethnographic methodologic assessment of pain perceptions by verbal description. *Pain, 34*(2), 195-204.

Muraki, E. (1992). A generalized partial credit model - Application of an EM algorithm. *Applied Psychological Measurement, 16*(2), 159-176.

National Institutes of Health. (2002). NIH State-of-the-Science Statement on symptom management in cancer: pain, depression, and fatigue. *NIH Consens State Sci Statements, 19*(4), 1-29.

Nikolaus, T., and Zeyfang, A. (2004). Pharmacological treatments for persistent non-malignant pain in older persons. *Drugs and Aging, 21*(1), 19-41.

Ohayon, M. M., and Schatzberg, A. F. (2003). Using chronic pain to predict depressive morbidity in the general population. *Archives of General Psychiatry, 60*(1), 39-47.

Portenoy, R. K., Thaler, H. T., Kornblith, A. B., Lepore, J. M., Friedlander-Klar, H., Kiyasu, E., et al. (1994). The Memorial Symptom Assessment Scale: an instrument for the evaluation of symptom prevalence, characteristics and distress. *European Journal of Cancer, 30A*(9), 1326-1336.

Portenoy, R. K., Ugarte, C., Fuller, I., and Haas, G. (2004). Population-based survey of pain in the United States: differences among white, African American, and Hispanic subjects. *Journal of Pain, 5*(6), 317-328.

Samejima, F. (1969). Estimation of latent ability using a response pattern of graded scores. *Psychometrika Monograph*, No. 17.

Samejima, F. (1972). A general model for free-response data. *Psychometrika Monograph*, No. 18.

Saunders, C. (1959). *The care of the dying*. London: Macmillan.

Schott, G. D. (2004). Communicating the experience of pain: the role of analogy. *Pain, 108*(3), 209-212.

Sheehan, D. C., and Forman, W. B. (1997). Symptomatic management of the older person with cancer. *Clinics in Geriatric Medicine, 13*(1), 203-219.

Singer, P. A., Martin, D. K., and Kelner, M. (1999). Quality end-of-life care: patients' perspectives. *Journal of the American Medical Association, 281*(2), 163-168.

Spiegel, D., Sands, S., and Koopman, C. (1994). Pain and depression in patients with cancer. *Cancer, 74*(9), 2570-2578.

Steinhauser, K. E., Clipp, E. C., McNeilly, M., Christakis, N. A., McIntyre, L. M., and Tulsky, J. A. (2000). In search of a good death: observations of patients, families, and providers. *Annals of Internal Medicine, 132*(10), 825-832.

Stiefel, F., and Stagno, D. (2004). Management of insomnia in patients with chronic pain conditions. *CNS Drugs, 18*(5), 285-296.

Strang, P. (1998). Cancer pain--a provoker of emotional, social and existential distress. *Acta Oncologica, 37*(7-8), 641-644.

Sutton, L. M., Porter, L. S., and Keefe, F. J. (2002). Cancer pain at the end of life: a biopsychosocial perspective. *Pain, 99*(1-2), 5-10.

Syrjala, K. L., and Chapko, M. E. (1995). Evidence for a biopsychosocial model of cancer treatment-related pain. *Pain, 61*(1), 69-79.

Thissen, D., Steinberg, L., and Wainer, H. (1988). Use of item response theory in the study of group differences in trace lines. In H. Wainer and H. I. Braun (Eds.), *Test validity*. Hillsdale, NJ: Lawrence Erlbaum Associates, Publishers.

Thurston, R. C., Keefe, F. J., Bradley, L., Rama Krishnan, K. R., and Caldwell, D. S. (2001). Chest pain in the absence of coronary artery disease: a biopsychosocial perspective. *Pain, 93*(2), 95-100.

Truchon, M. (2001). Determinants of chronic disability related to low back pain: towards an integrative biopsychosocial model. *Disability and Rehabilitation, 23*(17), 758-767.

Turk, D. C., and Monarch, E. S. (2002). Biopsychosocial perspective on chronic pain. In D. C. Turk and R. J. Gatchel (Eds.), *Psychological approaches to pain management: A practitioner's handbook* (2nd ed., pp. 3-29). New York: Guilford Press.

Wainer, H., Dorans, N. J., Flaugher, R., Green, B. F., Mislevy, R. J., Steinberg, L., et al. (Eds.). (2000). *Computerized adaptive testing: A primer* (2nd ed.). Mahwah, NJ: Lawrence Erlbaum Associates, Publishers.

Wainer, H., Dorans, N. J., Green, B. F., Steinberg, L., Flaugher, R., Mislevy, R. J., et al. (1990). *Computerized adaptive testing: A primer*. Hillsdale, NJ: Lawrence Erlbaum Assocaites, Publishers.

Weiss, D. J. (1982). Improving measurement quality and efficiency with adaptive theory. *Applied Psychological Measurement, 6*(4), 473-492.

Weiss, D. J. (1985). Adaptive testing by computer. *Journal of Consulting and Clinical Psychology, 53*(6), 774-789.

Weiss, D. J., and Kingsbury, G. (1984). Application of computerized adaptive testing to educational problems. *Journal of Educational Measurement, 21*(4), 361-375.

Yun, Y. H., Heo, D. S., Lee, I. G., Jeong, H. S., Kim, H. J., Kim, S. Y., et al. (2003). Multicenter study of pain and its management in patients with advanced cancer in Korea. *Journal of Pain and Symptom Management, 25*(5), 430-437.

Zimmerman, L., Story, K. T., Gaston-Johansson, F., and Rowles, J. R. (1996). Psychological variables and cancer pain. *Cancer Nursing, 19*(1), 44-53.

In: New Directions in Aging Research
Editor: Ruby R. Brougham, pp. 91-117
ISBN 978-1-60741-976-1
© 2009 Nova Science Publishers, Inc.

Chapter 6

Health Literacy and Older Adults: Understanding Cognitive and Emotional Barriers

Lisa Sparks[*2] *and Ruby R. Brougham*[1]
Chapman University, Department of Psychology, Orange, California, USA
Chao Family Comprehensive/NCI Designated Cancer Center,
University of California, Irvine, California, USA

Abstract

The current chapter reviews the relationship between health literacy, cognition, and emotion in older adults. Health literacy includes the concepts of accessing and understanding health information and services, with a comprehensive skill set of literacy that potentially includes visual (graphs and charts), computer (operate and search), information (obtain and apply relevant information), and numeracy (calculate and reason numerically) skills required to make appropriate health decisions. Current reports from the American Medical Association suggest that older adults, those over the age of 65, are the most vulnerable to the health consequences caused by poor health literacy. Older adults who have low health literacy are likely to have difficulty describing symptoms, providing an accurate health history, and understanding the health diagnosis and treatment recommended by their health care provider. Individuals with low health literacy have also been found to have greater medical expenditures in part attributable to a greater number of hospitalizations and the use of emergency room services, and medication nonadherence. The current chapter identifies and discusses the cognitive and emotional changes that impact information processing, communication, and decision-making. A specific research agenda for the study of older adults with low health literacy is provided.

* Correspondence concerning this article should be addressed to Lisa Sparks, Chapman University, Department of Psychology, Orange, California 92866 Electronic mail may be sent to sparks@chapman.edu

Introduction

One of the greatest challenges facing America in the 21st Century is the aging of the population. By 2030, the number of Americans over 65 will have more than doubled to 71.5 million, about 20% of the population (Federal Interagency Forum on Aging, 2008). Current reports suggest that older adults, those over 65 years of age, are the most vulnerable to the health consequences caused by poor health literacy (American Medical Association Foundation and American Medical Association, 2006; DeWalt, Berkman, Sheridan, Lohr, and Pignone, 2004; Paasche-Orlow, Schillinger, Greene, and Wagner, 2006; White, 2008; Wolf, Gazmararian, and Baker, 2005).

Health literacy is an important construct for understanding patients' needs for health information, as well as their abilities to access and utilize such health information and messages for critical health decision-making. Health literacy as defined by Healthy People 2010 is "the degree to which individuals have the capacity to obtain, process and understand basic health information and services needed to make appropriate health decisions that may affect the health of Americans and the ability of the healthcare system to provide effective, high quality care," (United States Department of Health and Human Services, 2000, chapter 11, page 20). As such, patients need to be able to competently evaluate and locate health information for credibility and quality, analyze relative risks and benefits, calculate dosages, interpret test results, etc. Health literacy includes the concepts of accessing and understanding information and services, with a comprehensive skill set of literacy that potentially includes visual (graphs and charts), computer (operate and search), information (obtain and apply relevant information), and numeracy (calculate and reason numerically) skills required to make appropriate health decisions (see e.g. Nielsen-Bohlman, Panzer, and Kindig, 2004; Ratzan, Lesar, and Filerman, 2000). Further, patients need strong oral communication skills to adequately and accurately describe their symptoms concerns, and to be able to competently search for and understand health information and make informed decisions. According to the American Medical Association (2006), poor health literacy is a better indicator of a person's health than demographic information, such as age, income, race and employment status (Ad Hoc Committee on Health Literacy for the Council on Scientific Affairs, American Medical Association, 1999). Nielsen-Bohlman, Panzer, and Kindig (2004) report that ninety million people in the United States, nearly half the population, have difficulty understanding and using health information. As a result, patients often take medicines on erratic schedules, miss follow-up appointments, and do not understand instructions like "take on an empty stomach".

Health literacy indicates the extent to which and individual has the ability to communicate verbally, familiarity and comprehension of technical health and science information, navigating the health care system, and relational agency (O'Hair and Sparks, 2008) among others. Education, culture, ethnicity and race, family, health status, and numerous other factors potentially influence being able to obtain, process, and understand information. Health literacy appears to be an important factor for health care knowledge, usage, screening rates and medication adherence, (Davis, Williams, Marin, Parker, and Glass, 2002; Davis, et al., 2006; Kreps and Sparks, 2008; Sparks and Nussbaum, 2008).

Older adults have been found to have low health literacy rates. White (2008) reports from the National Assessment of Adult literacy (2003) that 59% of adult participants 65 and older had limited health literacy. The health literacy rates of older adults were also found to be lower than those of young and middle-age individuals (White, 2008). Furthermore, Rudd, Kirsch, and Yamamoto (2004) report that the health literacy of older adults was below average and that older adults have difficulty in many health literacy tasks, such as comprehending prescription instructions that include any level of complexity. Furthermore, Benson and Forman (2002) found that 30% of well-educated older adults had difficulty with comprehension of written materials.

Older adults are more likely than younger and middle age adults to suffer from chronic diseases (e.g., cancer, cardiovascular and diabetes) and more likely to use prescription medicines (Goulding, 2005; Kaufman, Kelly, Rosenberg, Anderson and Mitchell, 2002; Meltzer, 2008). Thus, older adults are more likely to interact frequently with the health care professionals and the health care system. Older adults who have low health literacy are likely to have difficulty describing symptoms, providing an accurate health history, and understanding the health diagnosis and treatment recommended by their health care provider. Past research has found that older people have difficult in comprehending medical information (Davis, et al., 2006; Morrell, Park and Poon, 1989). Patients and their family members need a complex set of health literacy skills to optimize the patient's treatment experiences. These skills include the ability to communicate, listen, remember appointments and instructions, ask for clarification, self-advocate, analyze risk factors and negotiate with insurers or health care providers (Kreps and Sparks, 2008; Kutner, Greenberg, Jin, and Paulsen, 2006; Nielsen-Bohlman, Panzer, and Kindig, 2004; Sparks and Nussbaum, 2008; Williams, Davis, Parker, and Weiss, 2002).

Thus, it is not surprising that American Medical Foundation and American Medical Association (2006) reports that 80% of medical errors are due to misunderstood health communications. Furthermore, individuals with low health literacy have been found to have greater medical expenditures in part attributable to a greater number of hospitalizations and the use of emergency room services, and medication nonadherence (Baker, et al., 2002; DeWalt, et al., 2004; Howard, Gazmararian, and Parker, 2005; MacLaughlin, et al., 2005; Paasche-Orlow, et al., 2006). Older adults with low levels of health literacy are also less likely to use preventive health services (such as flu shots and annual physical exams) and have greater difficulty in managing chronic health problems, and may also contribute to the increase need for hospitalization and emergency services (Sudore, et al., 2006; White, 2008).

The focus of this chapter is on the relationship between health literacy, cognition, and emotion in older adults. If we understand how cognition and emotion change in older adults, then we will have a better understanding of why older adults have reduced health literacy and how to design and communicate health materials for maximum effectiveness. The goals of this chapter are: 1) to review the cognitive and emotional changes in older adults that place them at greater risk for lower health literacy and impede health communication and decision-making and 2) to suggest strategies to improve health literacy among older adults. Specifically the current chapter will review: 1) reading, vision and cognitive abilities, 2) effortful and automatic processing, 3) spoken language comprehension, 4) decision-making, and 5) emotion. The chapter concludes with directions for future research including a discussion of the role of health care providers in improving health literacy in older adults and a specific research agenda.

Reading, Vision and Cognitive Abilities

Past studies suggest that reading level rather than years of education predicts health literacy levels (Institute of Medicine, 2004; Sudore, et al., 2006). People's performance on a general literacy (reading level) task and their performance on health literacy tasks are highly correlated (Baker, Gazmararian, Sudano, and Patterson, 2000; White, 2008). Poor reading skills may account for the use of television, radio, family and friends as primary sources of health information for individuals with low levels of health literacy (White, 2008).

Since reading requires the integration of vision, attention, working memory, and processing speed, the poor reading performance of older adults may reflect sensory and cognitive decline. Older adults experience the following age-related changes in vision: 1) require more light to see, 2) increased sensitivity to glare, 3) decreased ability to adapt to changes in illumination, 4) greater difficulty in seeing close objects or small print clearly (known as presbyopia), 5) difficulty in adapting vision from near to far objects, and 6) decreased ability to see detail and discriminate between patterns (know as visual acuity). Reading is likely to be particularly challenging when the print is small, single-space, and low in contrast, such as black text on a grey background. In addition, insufficient illumination and glare also contribute to making reading more difficult for the older person. Thus, age related changes in vision and lack of environmental accommodations (e.g., larger print) contribute to the decrease in reading performance of older adults (Aldwin and Gilmer, 2004; Hagerstrom-Portnoy and Morgan, 2006; Kline, 1994; Kline and Schreiber, 1985)

Age-related declines in the ability to perform cognitive tasks, such as reading, may be the result of decreased functioning of basic cognitive mechanisms. Specifically, decreased functioning of working memory, inhibition, and speed of processing has been posited to account for declines in cognitive functioning (Hasher and Zacks, 1988; Park and Schwarz, 2000; Salthouse, Hambrick, Lukas, and Dell, 1996). A brief description of each cognitive mechanism follows: 1) Working memory is the ability to temporarily store and process information often in conjunction with new incoming information (Baddeley, 1986; Zacks, Hasher, and Li, 2000); 2) Inhibition is the ability to focus on important information and ignore irrelevant information (Hasher and Zacks, 1988); and 3) Speed of processing is the rate at which cognitive operations are performed (Salthouse, et al., 1996). In general, as one ages there is a decline in the efficiency of these cognitive mechanisms. Overall, age related deficits in cognition are most pronounced when 1) a number of tasks must be completed simultaneously, 2) task complexity is high, and 3) the task is unfamiliar (Cerella and Hale, 1994; Chen, Hale, and Myerson, 2003; Kliegel and Martin, 2007). There is some debate as to whether age declines are due to: 1) a reduction in available cognitive resources for performing a task, 2) a decline in processing speed for performing a task, or 3) a decline in the ability to focus on a task and inhibit irrelevant information when performing a task (Craik and Byrd, 1982; Hasher and Zacks, 1988; Salthouse, 1991).

Deficits in the cognitive abilities of older adults also limit their retention of information (Park and Jones, 1996), comprehension and reasoning (Salthouse, 1992; Salthouse, 2000), and their ability to make inferences (Hancock, Rogers, and Fisk, 2001; Rogers, Rousseau, and Lamson, 1999). For example, Wilson and Park (2008) found that older adults remember the main idea of a sentence rather than the contextual details, such as whether the sentence is positive or negative. This deficit has important implication for communicating medical information. For example, medical information such as, "Exercising joints that are inflamed from arthritis is not harmful" is likely to be remembered by the older person as, "Exercising joints that are inflamed from arthritis is harmful." Older adults may have more difficult with the processing of negative information because it requires greater cognitive resources than positive information (Lea and Mulligan, 2002; MacDonald and Just, 1989). Hancock, Rogers and Fisk (2001) also found that older adults had difficulty in comprehending warning symbols on household products and over-the-counter medications. The comprehension of a warning symbol also places greater demand on cognitive resources because it requires the older adult to make an inference.

As evident by the preceding discussion, reading skills are dependent on vision and cognitive resources. Since written health materials have become a primary way to communicate health information (United States Department of Health and Human Services, 2000), age-related declines in vision and cognition place older adults at greater risk for ineffective health communication. Older adults often receive instruction about medical conditions, treatments, medications, side effects and preventive health care (e.g., vaccination for influenza) through written text, such as instructional and informational pamphlets. Clearly, effective health management requires accurate comprehension and memory of written text.

Designing written health care materials that address age-related changes in vision and cognition would facilitate communication between the health care provider and the older adult. The following guidelines provide recommendations for written materials that are informed by the research on age-related declines in vision and cognition: 1) avoid the use of complicated text and medical jargon (Bernier, 1993; Safeer and Keenan, 2005), 2) use a succinct and focused presentation of ideas (Jacobson, et al., 1999), 3) avoid negatively worded items, such as, "Do not stop taking your antibiotic when you feel better" instead use, "When you feel better continue taking your medication, until you finish all of your medication (Wilson and Park, 2008) 4) avoid the simultaneous discussion or presentation of multiple ideas, for example, the effects of a medication and the common side effects of a medication should be discussed in separate sections within an informational pamphlet (Mayeaux, et al., 1996; Parker, 2000), 5) the use of list rather than paragraphs (Morrow, Leirer, Andrassy, Hier, and Menard, 1998) 6) avoid symbols (Hancock, Rogers and Fisk, 2001) 7) use a large font size (Aldridge, 2004; Mayeaux, et al., 1996), 8) double-space all text (Anderson, Heibert, Scott, and Wilkinson, 1985; Doak, Doak, and Root, 1996), 9) do not use condensed text (Anderson, Heibert, Scott, and Wilkinson, 1985; Doak, Doak, and Root, 1996), and 10) maximize the contrast between text and background, for example use black text on a white background (Mayeaux, et al., 1996).

Although the greater experience and large knowledge base of older adults can reduce some of the impact of declining cognitive resources (e.g., Mireles and Charness, 2002) reading remains an activity that requires a substantial amount of cognitive resources. However, for certain health related activities, such as medication adherence for the long-term management of chronic health conditions, the experience of older adults has been found to have positive benefits in reducing medication errors (Park, et al., 1999). Park and Hall-Gutchess (2000) suggest that with time, practice, and cues from the everyday environment, the medication adherence behavior of older adults can became an automatic behavior that requires few cognitive resources. Thus, transforming an effortful task into an automatic task successfully reduces the amount of cognitive resources needed to complete the task. The next section of this chapter discusses effortful and automatic processing and their relationship to health literacy.

Effortful and Automatic Processing

An effortful task, such as learning to use a medical device, requires a substantial amount of cognitive resources. For example, an older adult learning to use a medical device employs 1) working memory to hold and manipulate new information, 2) long-term memory for retrieval of relevant information, 3) sustained attention for concentration, and 4) comprehension and general knowledge to solve problems as they occur. Past research shows that the ability to perform effortful tasks declines with age (Park, 1999). In particular, memory tasks that are unsupported by environmental cues are particularly challenging for older adults (Park and Jones, 1996). For example, older adults who were trained to use a complex medical device that involved several procedural steps would find it difficult after one training session to use the device. However, if older adults were provided with the appropriate environmental support, such as demonstration and review of task sequence and taught a memory strategy (e.g., mnemonic device) they would be more likely to remember the procedural steps involved in using the device. Past research suggest that in older adults the use of mnemonic devices aids memory (Brehmer, et al., 2008; O'Hara, et al., 2007), increasing structure and organization also aids memory and comprehension (Cavallini, Pagnin, and Vecchi, 2003; Morrow and Leirer, 1999), and simplifying text and adding picture aids in comprehension even when material is complicated, such as understanding advanced medical directives (Kools, van de Wiel, Ruiter, and Kok, 2006; Zwahr, Park, Eaton, and Larson, 1997).

In contrast to effortful processing, automatic processing is fast and reliable. When an effortful task is rehearsed the task eventually becomes automatic and requires few cognitive resources. Once the task is automatic it becomes a response to a specific stimulus and occurs without intention, for example, a person who has learned to ice skate is no longer conscious of the adjustments they make to balance on the ice skates.

Automatic processing, unlike effortful processing, does not show age related declines (Jacoby, Jennings, and Hay, 1996; Park and Hall-Gutchess, 2000). Thus, Brown and Park (2002) suggest that one means of improving health related behaviors in older people, such as medication compliance, is to automate the behavior. For example, the older person eats dinner and then takes her/his medication. Over time the process of taking medication becomes automatic. The act of eating dinner provides the stimulus for the automatic response of taking the medication. In support of automating behavior, Liu and Park (2004) found that older adults could be trained to use implementation intentions that facilitate the automazation of self-care health tasks. Furthermore, the automated response could be sustained over time. Creating an implementation intention consisted of visualizing the health related event and the cues that would be used in the environment. Implementation intentions are an easy to learn technique and have been successful in improving medication adherence where broader cognitive training for improving memory in everyday activities has met with less success (Ball, et al., 2002). In a clinical setting, a nurse or physician assistant could instruct the older adult on the process of forming an implementation intention before they leave the medical office and could follow-up with the older adult a few days later. Teaching implementation intention techniques is one means to addresses the issue of cognitive declines when delivering health care services to older adults.

As a result of hearing loss, spoken language comprehension may also become an effortful task, requiring older adults to expend their cognitive resources to discriminate sounds and thus reduce the available resources for memory and comprehension (Rabbit, 1990). The loss of hearing places the older adult at high risk for miscommunication in health care encounters. The next section of this chapter discusses the relationship between hearing, cognitive abilities, and health literacy.

Spoken Language Comprehension

Spoken language comprehension involves the integration of cognitive and sensory abilities. To understand the spoken word the listener must able to recognize words, determine the relationship between words, and properly interpret the meaning of the words (Wingfield, 2000). This can be challenging since the rate of speech is often quick between 140 to 180 wpm and people often under articulate sounds making it difficult to decipher words. Often the under articulation of words is not conscious and may be a result of greater familiarity with words in a particular context.

The National Institute on Deafness and Other Communication Disorders (2001) reports that the rate of hearing loss is about 33% in older adults (age 65 to 75). For those adults over 75, the rate of hearing loss is estimated at 50%. In particular, older adults suffer from presbycusis. One common symptom of presbycusis is difficulty in distinguishing higher-pitched sounds. Thus, it is difficult for the older individual to hear high frequency and low energy sounds such as *ch*, *sh*, *s*, and *th* and to discriminate between the sounds (National Institute on Deafness and Other Communication Disorders, 2001; Wingfield, 2000). In addition older adults may also suffer from phonemic regression, sounds may be unintelligible and the speech of others may seem mumbled or slurred. Thus, older adults with presbycusis will find it difficult to hear a conversation in the presence of background noise (Bertoli, Smurzynksi, and Probst, 2005). Furthermore, a decline in the rate at which attentional focus can be changed from one stimulus to another in combination with a decreased ability to sustain attentional focus may also make it more difficult for the older adult to separate speech from background noise (Tun, O'Kane and Wingfield, 2002). Since linguistic knowledge does not show age related declines, older adults have been found to rely on context more often than younger adults to fill in what they have missed in a conversation (Pichora-Fuller, Schneider, and Daneman, 1995). However, this compensation strategy may reduce the available cognitive resources for processing information. Thus, by using effortful processing to understand speech, the older person has less available resources to encode the information for memory or devote attentional resources to comprehending complicated messages, such as medical instructions (Schneider and Pichora-Fuller, 2000; Tun, O'Kane, Wingfield, 2002).

Hearing loss has also been associated with older adults' reports of a reduced quality of life (Dalton, et al., 2003). Reduction in older adults' quality of life may in part be attributable to an increased difficult in communicating with others. Communication difficulties result in fewer exchanges of information and conversations may be avoided due to hearing loss (Dalton, et al., 2003; Nussbaum, Pecchioni, Robinson, and Thompson, 2000). Isolation or decreased contact with family and friends may results in fewer chances to exercise communication skills and contribute to further decline of communication skills. Thus, people interacting with the older adult with the hearing loss may find communication to be difficult and challenging.

Past research suggests that individuals with low health literacy often rely heavily on verbal instructions from their health care provider (Baker, et al., 1996; Davis, et al., 2001; Shohet and Renaud, 2006). Thus, the dominant channel of communication, verbal instructions, will be obstructed for older adults who are experiencing hearing loss and cognitive declines. Thus, the older adult is less likely to find interactions with health care professionals as understandable or empowering (Baker, et al., 1996; Wolf, et al., 2007).

The health literacy of older persons who are experiencing hearing loss and declines in cognition can be improved by active approaches to health education. For example, in the "teach-back" technique the older adult is instructed on a medical procedure and then asked to teach the technique to the medical provider. In addition, speaking slowly, limiting the amount of information, and repeating information are also useful techniques for increasing the likelihood that the older adult will comprehend verbal medical instructions (Paasche-Orlow, Schillinger, Greene, and Wagner, 2006; Parker, 2000).

Clearly changes in sensory perception (hearing and vision) and declining cognitive processing result in greater difficulty for the older person in obtaining, processing, and understanding health care information. An additional problem for older adults is that they are often required to make decisions based on their understanding of health care information. Thus, the older person due to declines in sensory and cognitive processing may make an important health decision, such as choice of medical procedure, based upon insufficient information and a misunderstanding of the cost and benefits of a medical procedure. The next section of this chapter discusses the relationship between aging, health literacy, and decision-making.

Decision-Making

The lower health literacy of older adults places them at risk for poor health decision-making. As suggested in the National Assessment of Adult literacy (2003) study, older adults are often required to make decisions about following three broad types of health tasks: 1)

Clinical (e.g., diagnosis, treatment, and medication), 2) prevention (maintaining and improving health), and 3) navigation (e.g., understanding the rights and responsibilities associated with health care). Thus, older adults who are unable to comprehend health related information might fail to make appropriate decisions regarding several aspects of their health care.

Decision-making involves both a process and an outcome. The decision process of older adults shows some decline when compared to younger adults. Research studies suggest that in a variety of decision domains older adults need more time to make a decision, use less information, reason less, make fewer comparative judgments among alternatives, have greater difficulty understanding information about alternatives, have difficulty remembering alternatives, and are more likely to avoid a decision than younger adults (Chen and Sun, 2003; Finucane, et al., 2002; Finucane, Mertz, Solvic and Schmidtt, 2005; Hershey, Jacobs-Lawson, and Walsh, 2003; Johnson and Drungle, 2000; Mata, Schooler, and Reiskamp, 2007; Meyer, Russo and Talbot, 1995; Sanfey and Hastie, 2000; Walsh and Hershey, 1993; Wood, Busemeyer, Koling, Cox, and Davis, 2005; Zwahr, et al., 1997). Older adults also make less effective decisions when situations are novel and time constrained (Finucane, et al., 2002; Johnson, 1990; Mata, Schooler, and Rieskamp, 2007; Sanfey and Hastie, 2000). Although older adults continue to be adaptive in matching their decision strategies with the demands of a task, they more often rely on simpler decisions strategies than younger adults (Mata, Schooler, and Reiskamp, 2007). However, the final outcome of the decision process is often similar for young and older adults (Finucane, et al., 2002; Hershey, Jacobs-Lawson, and Walsh, 2003; Meyer, Russo and Talbot, 1995; Walsh and Hershey, 1993; Zwahr, et al., 1997). Thus, the decision-making process of older adults shows deficits in effortful processing.

Since age related declines in decision-making are found for effortful processing but not for decisions that require less cognitive processing, such as decisions that are familiar, without time constraint, and are adequately addressed with simple decision strategies it is likely that older adults would benefit from decision strategies that reduce cognitive processing. Shared decision making with a health care professional is one strategy that has the potential for reducing the cognitive demands of a health decision. Shared decision-making consists of communication and participation from both health care provider and patient in making decisions about health care. However, in order for shared decision making to be effective the health care professional must be able to clearly outline the health decision. Specifically, the health care provider should communicate the objectives of the health decision, the alternatives, the consequences, the risks, and assist the older person in understanding the trade-offs or compromises that will need to be made. For example, in deciding whether to take a recommended medication the older adult needs to understand clearly what is the objective of the medication, that is, what is likely to change as a result of taking the medication? The cost and benefits of the medication and clear identification of the risks involved with taking the medication must also be provided. The health care provider may have a tendency to focus on the disease-specific outcomes, such as a decrease in cholesterol. Patients, however, are more likely to focus on inconvenience, cost, side effects, such as impaired physical and cognitive functioning and also time to expected benefits (Dickinson and Raynor, 2003; Lewis, Robinson and Wikinson, 2003). Thus, a discussion of compromise for the agreed upon course of medical action is necessary to provide a medical outcome that is acceptable to both the older adult and health care provider. A main advantage of shared decision-making is that the health care provider and older adult share information. Thus, the values and preferences of the older adult are known and used as important decision criteria for a health decision in combination with knowledge about risk and the cost and benefits related to the decision outcome to determine the best course of medical action.

Although shared decision-making is associated with improved health outcomes and greater adherence to medications (Corser, Holmes-Rovner, Lein, and Gossain, 2007; Mandelblatt, Kreling, Figeuriedo, and Feng, 2006), some older adults report a reluctance to participate in shared decision strategies (Arora, and McHorney, 2000; Levinson, Kao, Kuby, and Thisted, 2005). Some older adults prefer a paternalistic model of health care where health decisions are completely determined by the health care provider (Elkin, Kim, Casper, Kissane, and Schrag, 2007; Flynn, Smith, and Vanness, 2006). However, other barriers such as poor communication, lack of trust, fear, lack of knowledge, and low self-esteem have been cited by older adults as reasons for not participating in shared decision-making (Belcher, Fried, Agostini, and Tinetti, 2006; Elkin, et al., 2007). Past research also suggest that the inability of older adults to articulate clear health goals is another obstacle to shared decision-making (Belcher, et al., 2006; Epstein, Alper and Quill, 2004; Schulman-Green, Naik, McCorkle, Bradley, and Bogardus, 2005). Schulman-Green, et al. (2005) propose that one way to facilitate shared decision making with older adults is through identifying the value they place on health and setting goals for health outcomes. Goal setting has been found to increase compliance to physician recommendations (Bogardus, et al., 2004; Corser, et al., 2007; Naik, Kallen, Walder, and Street, 2008) and increase progress toward health goals (Nothwehr and Yang, 2007). Schulman-Green, et al. (2005) suggests that goal setting facilitates communication between health care provider and older adult. Specifically, goal setting allows older adults the opportunity to identify and communicate important values and preferences to their health care provider and this communication provides the foundation for an individualized or tailored health plan that has support from both the older adult and health care provide. Furthermore, since goal setting engenders greater communication between health care provider and older adult and increases the commitment from the older adult to the mutually agreed upon goals of treatment, it is likely that health outcomes within the control of the older adult, such as management of chronic disease are likely to improve.

As suggested by Ford, Shofield, and Hope (2003) it is important that there be a match between the roles that adults desire in the health care decisions and the roles that they are offered. Past research has found that higher education, greater cognitive ability, less serious illness, being a woman, and younger age were associated with greater preference for increased participation in health decisions (Flynn and Smith, 2007; Flynn, Smith, and Vanness, 2006; Kaplan, et al., 1995; Petrisek, Laliberte, Allen and Mor, 1997). Flynn, Smith and Vanness (2006) also found that older adults were not passive participants in health care decisions, however, they did show great variability in their desired level of involvement, particularly in discussing and in making health care decisions (Flynn, Smith, and Vanness, 2006). Older adults with less education were found to be interested in high information exchange, that is, they were willing to provide a complete medical history to their physician and wanted to be fully informed regarding all of their health care options. However, they were less likely desire participation in the final decision for the choice of treatment. Thus, older adults with low literacy would benefit from tailoring shared decision-making to meet their needs for: 1) education, including explanation of risks and benefits and identification of alternative courses of action, 2) communication, including goals, values and preferences, and 3) decision-making, including an agreed upon course of medical action.

The previous discussion of decision-making has primarily focused on cognition; however, emotion also plays an important role in decision-making. For example, Loewenstein, Hsee, Weber and Welch (2001) propose that emotion, particular as expressed in reaction to risk can override cognition and become the dominant motivation for decision-making. The following chapter will discuss the relationship between emotion, aging, and health literacy.

Emotion, Aging and Health Literacy

The past discussion has focused on how declines in sensory and cognitive processing of older adults result in greater problems with health literacy. In contrast, emotional processing and emotional regulation do not show age related declines and may improve in older age (Charles, Mather, and Cartensen, 2003). Emotional processing tends to be fast and automatic, while cognitive processing is slow, deliberate, controlled and effortful. For example, Slovic, Finucane, Peters and MacGregor, (2002) suggest that people are guided by an affective heuristic that allows people under conditions of stress or cognitive overload to process information guide by fast, intuitive, emotional processes. Thus, emotional processing requires fewer cognitive resources and responses can be made quickly.

It is well documented that older adults show the following processing biases for emotion: 1) they report less negative affect (Carstensen, Pasupathi, Mayr, and Nesselroade, 2000), 2) they are more likely to pay attention to and remember positive information (Charles, Mather and Carstensen, 2003; Mather and Carstensen, 2003; Sullivan, Ruffman, and Hutton, 2007), and 3) they have greater difficulty recognizing negative emotions, such as anger, sadness and fear (Isaacowitz, et al., 2007). The age related shift that occurs away from the dominant use and processing of negative information in youth is known as the positivity effect (Carstensen and Mikels, 2005). Socioemotional selectivity theory is offered as an explanation for the age-related changes in motivation and the cognitive processing of emotional information (Carstensen, 1995; Carstensen, Isaacowitz and Charles, 1999). Socioemotional selectivity theory posits that older adults place greater value on emotionally meaningful goals as a result of a shorten future time perspective, the recognition of their time as limited, thus greater cognitive resources are used to obtain emotionally meaningful goals.

Emotions can influence the health care decisions and health actions of older adults. In particular, decisions that involve risk are most likely to evoke emotion. Emotions can play an informational role in decision-making, they can help people to evaluate alternative course of actions. However, for older adults with low health literacy emotional reactions may be more pronounced due to an increase in anxiety over understanding and evaluating health information. For example, fear has been found to make people more risk averse (Lerner, Gonzales, Small, and Fischhoff, 2003; Lerner and Keltner, 2001) thus a woman who is afraid to find out the results of a mammography may decide to forgo the preventive screening. The woman is experiencing dread; an emotion defined as feeling lack of control, fear, and anxiety (Peters and Slovic, 1996). Furthermore, anxiety increases people's preference for low risk, low reward options (Maner and Schmidt, 2006; Raghunathan and Pham, 1999). Thus, increased anxiety may account for the poorer decision-making skills of older individuals with low health literacy. Older adults with low health literacy may find interactions with health care providers and the health care system to be stressful (Sparks and Nussbaum, 2008). Stress is also related to having greater negative affect (Mroczek and Almeida, 2004; Zautra, Affleck, Tennen, Reich, and Davis, 2005). In past studies, negative affect has been associated with greater pessimism in judgment and choices (Lerner and Keltner, 2000). Thus, the older adult may be more likely to make choices that are risk averse as a result of negative affect. Health decisions that avoid risk are not always the best decisions.

Medical decision making often involves making decision that are personally relevant and have high stakes in terms of personal consequences, such as deciding whether to undergo chemotherapy treatment for cancer, and thus these decisions are likely to provoke a strong emotional response. The risk-as-feelings hypothesis (Loewenstein, et al., 2001) proposes that people's responses to risky situations are in part the result of emotions that are not cognitively processed. Neurological evidence supports this hypothesis. Specifically, LeDoux (1996) found that are direct neural projections from the thalamus to the amygdala that allow for instant emotional reaction to sensory information without cognitive processing. Since feelings and cognitive evaluations of risk are influenced by different factors, conflict often arises between cognitive and emotion, thus people's subsequent behavior may not follow the best course of action. For example, changes in probability, such as making it highly unlikely that one decision alternative would occur, results in changing the person's cognitive evaluation of the decision but not the person's feelings about the decision.

Anticipatory emotions also play a role in decision-making. Loewenstein and Lerner (2003) suggests that the emotions that people expect to experience as a result of making a particular choice influences their decision-making. For example, an older person trying to decide whether to undergo a medical procedure might imagine the regret she/he would feel if they agree to the medical procedure and it was unsuccessful. Vividness, the ability to imagine a decision outcome, evokes strong emotional reactions (Nisbett and Ross, 1980). Focusing on feelings and the use of mental imagery to image future consequences impacts people's decision-making in risky situations (Shiv, and Huber, 2000; van Dijk, van Roosmalen, Otten, and Stalmeier, 2008). Personal experience also has been found to modify people's emotional reactions to risk, in some situations making them more risk adverse and in other situations making them more risk seeking (Weinstein, 1989). For example, women's moderate experience of worry about breast cancer increases mammography participation (Diefenbach, Miller and Daly, 1999). Some support also exists for worry and regret, as motivation for people to get a flu shot in a subsequent year after they had initially refused a flu shot (Chapman, and Coups, 2006). Thus, older adults may engage in preventive health behaviors in an effort to reduce feelings of worry and regret and maintain positive affect. However, high levels of anxiety are associated with avoidance of preventative health screenings (Andersen, Smith, Meischke, Bowen, and Urban, 2003).

The common sense model proposed by Leventhal, Difenbach, and Leventhal (1992) suggests that people's health decisions and behaviors are motivated by a desire to regulate health threats and emotional response. Since taking action or making health decision may evoke worry, dread or regret an older adult may decide to avoid making a decision or decision making in an effort to regulate emotions. This may be one way to avoid negative affect and maintain positive affect. Past research also suggests that older adults who endorse powerful others as controlling their lives are less likely to seek health related information (Koo, Krass, and Aslani, 2006) and more likely to report greater emotional well-being (Harris, Cook, Victor, DeWilde, and Beighton, 2006). Thus, in making medical decisions older adults are likely to allow someone else (e.g., physician) to make a health decision for them (Elkin, et al., 2007; Sparks and Turner, 2008; Steginga, Occhipinti, Gardiner, Yaxley, and Heathcote, 2002).

In contrast to anticipatory emotions (emotional forecasts of how one will feel in the future if certain outcomes occur) are immediate emotions (the emotions that people feel at the time of decision-making), such as fear regarding a medical procedure. Decisions that are driven by immediate emotions may appear impulsive and may conflict with the best course of action as assessed by careful processing of the costs and benefits of a decision (Loewenstein and Lerner, 2003).

Although our understanding of the relationship between health, aging, and emotion continues to develop, we can make the following clinical suggestions for health messages for older adults with low health literacy: 1) messages that appeal to emotion are more likely to be successful than those that are related to health statistics, and 2) messages that are positively framed (e.g., If you get a flu shot today, you are likely to be healthy this winter) are more likely to be attend to, processed and remembered by the older adult than messages that are negatively framed (e.g., If you do not get a flu shot today, it is unlikely that you will be healthy this winter), and 3) health decisions that are repeated, such as the decision to get a flu shot or a mammogram may be influenced by past emotions of worry and regret. Furthermore, older adults with low health literacy may be more prone to anxiety and stress in a health care situation and negatively framed health care messages (e.g., If you do not get a flu shot today, it is unlikely that you will be healthy this winter) may increase fear and arousal to high level and thus reduce the effectiveness of the health care interaction.

Although worry and regret have been shown to predict preventive behaviors such as cancer screening, contraception, flu shot (Chapman, and Coups, 2006; Diefenbach, Miller, and Daly, 1999; Moser, McCaul, Peters, Nelson, and Marcus, 2007; Richard, de Vries, and van der Pligt, 1998). The role of other emotions in health decision-making, in particular positive emotions is not well researched.

Conclusion

Recommendations for Future Research

Since older adults are the largest consumer of healthcare services (Cohen, Martinez, and Free, 2006) and as the baby boomer generation (those born between 1946 and 1964) begins to retire the number of older adults using health care services will increase (National Center for Health Statistics, 2003). The baby boom generation is a diverse population including many individuals who are healthier, have greater education, have greater wealth, and can expect greater longevity in retirement than past cohorts. However, this population also includes those who have few resources for retirement, chronic health problems, and low rates of education (Center for Health Communication, Harvard School of Public Health, 2004). One important challenge that we face is how to address the diversity of our older population and find methods to deliver quality health services to older adults with low health literacy.

Individuals with low health literacy of all ages share a common problem in difficulty with comprehension of health material (White, 2008). Comprehension is a critical skill that allows individuals to successfully engage in clinical (e.g., diagnosis, treatment, and medication), prevention (maintaining and improving health), and navigation (e.g., understanding the rights and responsibilities associated with health care) tasks. As discussed in this chapter, for the older adult difficulty in comprehending health material may be the result of declines in vision and cognitive abilities. One promising area of research for improving comprehension in low health literate adults is the use of pictures in written health materials (Houts, Doak, Doak, and Loscalzo, 2006; Houts, Witmer, Egeth, Loscalzo, and Zabora, 2001; Kripalani, et al., 2007). Although, many improvements have been made in text design for written health materials, such as the use of a large font size, fewer improvements have been made in text presentation, such as avoiding negatively worded sentences (e.g., Wilson and Park, 2008), and many of the text comprehension difficulties of older adults remain unaddressed. Since past research suggests that deficits in comprehension are related to deficits in memory and that both lack of comprehension and inability to recall information lead to reduced medical adherence (Morrell, Park and Poon, 1989; Park, Morrell, Frieske, and Kincaid, 1992), it is imperative that future research continues to identify ways to increase the comprehension of older adults with low literacy.

The baby boom generation (those born between 1946 and 1964) is more likely to access the Internet for health care information than previous generations. Past studies suggest that 72% of individuals age 50 - 64 subscribe to Internet service and 53% of this age group use the Internet for healthcare information (The American Consumer Institute, 2006; Dickerson, et al., 2004). Although text continues to be the dominant means for communicating health care information on-line, there has been some effort to use text in combination with graphics, videos and animation (Baur, 2005). For on-line healthcare information educational interactivity and user input have been identified as critical elements (Davis, et al., 1998). For example watching health care demonstrations of skills and then being able to practice and apply those skills has been found to be an effective means to communicate health care information (Echt, Morrell and Park, 1998). Thus, on-line presentation of health care materials may be one efficient means that allows the tailoring of healthcare information by providing specific and personalized healthcare recommendations. For example, in providing nutritional information the person's cultural background would be taken into account and used to present personalized recommendations for meal plans.

Delivering health care information to older adults with low health literacy using computer technology, such as the Internet is a relatively new research area that shows promise for increasing health literacy. Gerber, et al., (2005) found that although older adults with low health literacy were less likely to own a computer or to have computer experience but they still rated a computerized health intervention as "easy to use," however, they also used the health intervention program less than older people with higher health literacy. Kressig and Echt (2002) also found that older adults who rated a computerized exercise promotion program as easy to use were likely to accept the exercise recommendations of the program. Thus, there is some support for the use of computer technology as one means to increase the health literacy of older adults. Clearly, ease of use is one important consideration in designing computer programs to increase the health literacy of older adults. Another consideration is that older adults with poor health literacy may have less access to computers and less experience using computers. One potential solution is to have computer access in health care settings and to have a designated health care individual (e.g., nurse) who teaches the individual how to access information.

Health Care Providers

As the United States population continues to age, health care providers can play an important role in improving the health literacy of older adults. In the past, the dominant approach to health education has been a passive approach where the older adults is expected to read, understand, and act on health information with little assistance from health care providers (Parker, 2000). Current recommendations for improving health literacy involve interaction and the tailoring of health information (Davis, et al., 2006; Sparks and Turner, 2008). However, health care provider compliance with these recommendations may be a problem (Wright, Sparks, O'Hair, 2007). For example, Schwartzberg, Cowett, VanGeest, and Wolf (2007) found that although physicians, nurses, and pharmacists reported that techniques, such as using models or pictures to explain a medical concept, should be effective for increasing health literacy they seldom used the techniques (less than 50% of the time). The only strategies that were routinely used were simple language, avoiding medical jargon (95% of the time) and handing out printed materials to patients (70% of time). Thus, health care providers were more likely to use basic techniques that were easy to implement (such as using basic language) than more advanced techniques (such as teach-back technique) that were more difficult to implement and also required some training. Furthermore, Schwartzberg, et al. (2007) found that use of a particular technique by a health care provider to improve health literacy resulted in greater confidence in the technique and greater comfort in using the technique. Thus, education for health care providers is one method for improving compliance to health literacy recommendations. In particular, education that matches a specific clinical role is likely to be most effective. For example, physicians are likely to be engaged in making decisions with patients regarding health care, thus health literacy education for physicians should target shared decision-making and goal setting with patients. Although education increases knowledge and skills it does not address the other potential barriers to using techniques that will improve health literacy. Other barriers may include inconvenience, and lack of time, while other barriers may be more difficult to detect such as stereotypes about aging. Clearly, further research needs to 1) identify the barriers of health professionals in using health literacy techniques, and 2) continue to demonstrate the impact of using health literacy techniques on clinical outcomes (such as medical adherence and participation in preventive health screenings).

Research Agenda

A research agenda for improving the health literacy of older adults consists of the following: 1) improving accessibility of health care materials, this includes finding methods to enhancing readability of text through continued improvements in text design (e.g., larger type) and text presentation (e.g., using pictures to accompany text), 2) exploring new avenues for health care information and communication such as the Internet and e-mail, 3) exploring the effectiveness of multimedia presentation (text, photos, and videos) of health care information presented on the Internet, 4) continuing to find and test methods to enhance communication, such as shared decision-making and goal setting, between the older adult and health care provider, 5) continuing to improve older adults basic skill sets informed by research on cognitive and sensory changes in older adults, such as, implementation intentions that facilitate the automazation of self-care health tasks for older adults are the result of understanding declines in cognitive processes, 6) increasing the skills of health care providers and their use of effective techniques, such as using the teach-back technique, with older adults, 7) understanding and addressing the health professional barriers to using health literacy techniques, and 8) continued research on the role of emotion in health decision and use of that information to improve strategies for health literacy.

Many challenges continue to exist for the older adult with low health literacy. The future will bring an increasing number of older adults with diverse backgrounds and it will be imperative that we find efficient ways to communicate health information. As our understanding of cognitive, sensory (vision and hearing), and emotional processing of older adults increases we will be able to apply that knowledge to the domain of health literacy. Thus, the future of health literacy interventions for older adults holds great promise for effective strategies that are informed by research studies.

References

Ad Hoc Committee on Health Literacy for the Council on Scientific Affairs, American Medical Association. (1999). Health literacy: report of the Council on Scientific Affairs. *Journal of American Medical Association*, 281(6), 552-557.

Aldridge, M. D. (2004). Writing and designing readable patient education materials. *Nephrology Nursing Journal: Journal of the American Nephrology Nurses' Association, 31*(4), 373-377.

Aldwin, C. M., and Gilmer, D. F. (2004). *Health, illness, and optimal aging: Biological and psychosocial perspectives*. Thousand Oaks, CA: Sage Publishing.

American Medical Association Foundation and American Medical Association. (2006). *Health literacy: Safe communication universal precautions* (pp. 1-6). Chicago: American Medical Association.

Andersen, M. R., Smith, R., Meischke, H., Bowen, D., and Urban, N. (2003). Breast cancer worry and mammography use by women with and without a family history in a population-based sample. *Cancer Epidemiology, Biomarkers and Prevention, 12*, 314-320.

Anderson, R. C., Hiebert, E. H., Scott, J. A., and Wilkinson, I. A. G. (1985). *Becoming a nation of readers: The report of the commission on reading* (pp. 7-12). Champaign, IL: University of Illinois, Center for the Study of Reading; Washington, DC: National Institute of Education.

Arora, N. K., and McHorney, C. A. (2000). Patient preferences for medical decision making: Who really wants to participate? *Medical Care, 38*(3), 335-341.

Baddeley, A. (1986). *Working memory*. New York: Oxford University Press.

Baker, D. W., Gazmararian, J. A., Sudano, J., and Patterson, M. (2000). The association between age and health literacy among elderly persons. *The Journals of Gerontology, 55B*(6), S368-S374.

Baker, D. W, Gazmararian, J. A., Williams, M. V, Scott, T., Parker, R. M., Green, D., et al. (2002). Functional health literacy and the risk of hospital admission among Medicare managed care enrollees. *American Journal of Public Health, 92*(8), 1278-1283.

Baker, D. W., Parker, R. M., Williams, M. V., Pitkin, K., Parikh, N. S., Coates, W, et al. (1996). The health care experience with low literacy. *Archives of Family Medicine, 5*(6), 329-334.

Ball, K., Berch, D. B., Helmers, K. F., Jobe, J. B., Leveck, M. D., Marsiske, M., et al. (2002). Effects of cognitive training interventions with older adults: A randomized controlled trial. *The Journal of the American Medical Association, 288*(18), 2271-2281.

Baur, C. E. (2005). Using the Internet To Move Beyond the Brochure and Improve Health Literacy. In J. G. Schwartzberg, J. B. VanGeest, C. C. Wang (Eds.), *Understanding Health Literacy* (pp. 141-154). Chicago, IL: AMA Press

Belcher, V. N., Fried, T. R., Agostini, J. V., and Tinetti, M. E. (2006). Views of older adults on patient participation in medication-related decision making. *Journal of General Internal Medicine, 21*(4), 298-303.

Benson, J. G., and Forman, W. B. (2002). Comprehension of written health care information in an affluent geriatric retirement community: Use of the Test of Functional Health Literacy. *Gerontology, 48*(2), 93-97.

Bernier, M. J. (1993). Developing and evaluating printed education materials: A perspective model for quality. *Orthopaedic Nursing, 12*(6), 39-46.

Bertoli, S., Smurzynski, J., and Probst, R. (2005). Effects of age, age-related hearing loss and contralateral cafeteria noise on the discrimination of small frequency changes: Psychoacoustic and electrophysiological measures. *Journal of the Association for Research in Otolaryngology, 6*, 207-222.

Bogardus, S. T., Bradley, E. H., Williams, C. S., Maciejewski, P. K., Gallo, W. T., Inouye, S. K., et al. (2004). Achieving goals in geriatric assessment: Role of caregiver agreement and adherence to recommendations. *Journal of American Geriatric Society, 52*, 99-105.

Brehmer, Y., Li, S. C., Straube, B., Stoll, G., von Oertzen, T., Muller, V., et al. (2008). Comparing memory skill maintenance across the life span: Preservation in adults, increase in children. *Psychology and Aging, 23*(2), 227-238.

Brown, S. C., and Park, D. C. (2002). Roles of age and familiarity in learning health information. *Educational Gerontology, 28*, 695-710.

Carstensen, L. L. (1995). Evidence for a life span theory of socioemotional selectivity. *Current Directions in Psychological Science, 4*(5), 151-156.

Carstensen, L. L., Isaacowitz, D. M., and Charles, S. T. (1999). Taking time seriously: A theory of socioemotional selectivity. *American Psychologist, 54*(3), 165-181.

Carstensen, L. L., and Mikels, J. A. (2005). At the intersection of emotion and cognition: Aging and the positivity effect. *Current Directions in Psychological Science, 14*(3), 117-121.

Carstensen, L. L., Pasupathi, M., Mayr, U., and Nesselroade, J. R. (2000). Emotional experience in every life across adult life span. *Journal of Personality and Social Psychology, 79*, 644-655.

Cavallini, E., Pagnin, A., and Vecchi, T. (2003). Aging and everday memory: The beneficial effect of memory training. *Archives of Gerontology and Geriatrics, 37*(3), 241-257.

Center for Health Communication, Harvard School of Public Health. (2004). *Reinventing aging: Baby boomers and civic engagement.* Boston, MA: Harvard School of Public Health.

Cerella, J., and Hale, S. (1994). The rise and fall in information-processing rates over the life span. *Acta Psychologica*, 86(2-3), 109-197.

Chapman, G. B., and Coups, E. J. (2006). Emotions and preventative health behavior: Worry, regret, and influenza vaccination. *Health Psychology,* 25(1), 82-90.

Charles, S. T., Mather, M., and Carstensen, L. L. (2003). Aging and emotional memory: The forgettable nature of negative images for older adults. *Journal of Experimental Psychology: General, 132*, 310-324.

Chen, J., Hale, S., and Myerson, J. (2003). Effects of domain, retention interval, and information load on young and older adults' visuospatial working memory. *Aging Neuropsychology and Cognition, 10*(2), 122-133.

Chen, J., Hale, S., and Myerson, J. (2007) Predicting the size of individual and group differences on speeded cognitive tasks. *Psychonomic Bulletin and Review*, 14, 534-541.

Chen, Y., and Sun, Y. (2003). Age differences in financial decision-making: Using simple heuristics. *Educational Gerontology, 29*, 627-635.

Cohen, R. A., Martinez, M . E., and Free, H.L. (2006*). Health insurance coverage: Early release of estimates from the national health interview survey, January – September 2007* (CDC Division of Health Interview Statistics, National Center for Health Statistics). Washington, DC: Center for Disease Control and Prevention.

Corser, W., Holmes-Rovner, M., Lein, C., and Gossain, V. (2007). A shared decision-making primary care intervention for type 2 diabetes. *The Diabetes Educator, 33*(4), 700-708.

Craik, F. I. M., and Byrd, M. (1982). Aging and cognitive deficits: The role of attentional resources. In F. I. M. Craik and S. Trehub (Eds.), *Aging and cognitive processes* (pp. 191-211). New York: Plenum.

Dalton, D. S., Cruickshanks, K. J., Klein, B. E. K., Klein, R., Wiley, T. L., and Nondahl, D. M. (2003). The impact of hearing loss on quality of life in older adults. *The Gerontologist, 43*(5), 661-668.

Davis, T. C., Berkel, H. J., Arnold, C. L., Nandy, I., Jackson, R. H., and Murphy, P. W. (1998). Intervention to increase mammography utilization in a public hospital. *Journal of General Internal Medicine, 13*(4), 230-233.

Davis, T. C., Dolan, N. C., Ferreira, M. R., Tomori, C., Green, K. W., Sipler, A. M., et al. (2001). The role of inadequate health literacy skills in colorectal cancer screening. *Cancer Investigation, 19*(2), 193-200.

Davis, T. C., Williams, M. V., Marin, E., Parker, R. M., and Glass, J. (2002). Health literacy and cancer communication. *CA Cancer Journal for Clinicians, 52*, 134-154.

Davis, T. C., Wolf, M. S., Bass, P. F. III, Middlebrooks, M., Kennen, E., Baker, D. W., et al. (2006). Low literacy impairs comprehension of prescription drug warning labels. *Journal of General Internal Medicine, 21*, 847-851.

Davis, T. C., Wolf, M. S., Bass III, P. F., Thompson, J. A., Tilson, H. H., Neuberger, M, et al. (2006). Literacy and misunderstanding prescription drug labels. *Annals of Internal Medicine, 145*(12), 887-894.

DeWalt, D. A., Berkman, N. D., Sheridan, S., Lohr, K. N., and Pignone, M. P. (2004). Literacy and health outcomes: A systematic review of the literature. *Journal of General Internal Medicine, 13*, 1228-1239.

Dickerson, S., Reinhart, A. M., Feeley, T. H., Bidani, R., Rich, E., Garg, V. K., et al. (2004). Patient internet use for health information at three urban primary care clinics. *Journal of the American Medical Informatics Association, 11*(6), 499-504.

Dickinson, D., and Raynor, D. K. T. (2003). Ask the patients – they may want to know more than you think. *British Medical Journal, 327*(7419), 861-864.

Diefenbach, M. A., Miller, S. M., and Daly, M. B. (1999). Specific worry about breast cancer predicts mammography use in women at risk for breast and ovarian cancer. *Health Psychology, 18*, 532-536.

Doak, C. C., Doak, L. G., Root, J. H. (1996). *Teaching patients with low-literacy skills* (2nd ed). Philadelphia, PA: JB Lippincott Co.

Echt, K. V., Morrell, R. W., and Park, D. C. (1998). Effects of age and training formats on basic computer skill acquisition in older adults. *Educational Gerontology, 24*, 3-25.

Elkin, E. B., Kim, S. H. M., Casper, E. S., Kissane, D. W., and Schrag, D. (2007). Desire for information and involvement in treatment decisions: Elderly cancer patients' preferences and their physicians' perceptions. *Journal of Clinical Oncology: Official Journal of the American Society of Clinical Oncology, 25*(33), 5275-5280.

Epstein, R. M., Alper, B. S., and Quill, T. E. (2004). Communicating evidence for participatory decision making. *Journal of American Medical Association*, 291(19), 2359-2366.

Federal Interagency Forum on Aging-Related Statistics. (2008). Older Americans 2008: Key indicators of well-being. Washington, DC: Author.

Finucane, M. L., Mertz, C. K., Slovic, P., and Schmidt, E. S. (2005). Task complexity and older adults' decision-making competence. *Psychology and Aging, 20*(1), 71-84.

Finucane, M. L., Slovic, P., Hibbard, J., Peters, E., Mertz, C. K., MacGregor, D. G., et al. (2002). Aging and decision-making competence: An analysis of comprehension and consistency skills in older versus younger adults considering health plan options. *Journal of Behavioral Decision Making, 15*, 141-164.

Flynn, K. E., and Smith, M. A. (2007). Personality and health care decision-making style. *The Journals of Gerontology Series B: Psychological Sciences and Social Sciences, 62*, P261-P267.

Flynn, K. E., Smith, M., and Vanness, D. (2006). A typology of preference for participation in healthcare decision making. *Social Science and Medicine, 63*(5), 1158-1169.

Ford, S., Schofield, T., and Hope, T. (2003). Are patients' decision-making preferences being met? *Health Expectations: An international journal of public participation in health care and health policy, 6*(1), 72-80.

Gerber, B. S., Brodsky, I. G., Lawless, K. A., Smolin, L. I., Arozullah, A. M., Smith, E. V., et al. (2005). Implementation and evaluation of a low-literacy diabetes education computer multimedia application. *Diabetes Care, 28*(7), 1574-1580.

Goulding, M. R. (2005). Trends in prescribed medicine use and spending by older Americans, 1992-2001. *Aging Trends, No. 5.* Hyattsville, Maryland: National Center for Health Statistics.

Hagerstrom-Portnoy, G., and Morgan, M. (2006). Normal age-related vision changes. In A. J. Rosenbloom (Ed.) *Rosenbloom and Morgan's vision and aging* (pp. 31-48). St. Louis, MI : Butterworth-Heinemann

Hancock, H. E., Rogers, W. A., and Fisk, A. D. (2001). An evaluation of warning habits and beliefs across the adult life span. *Human Factors, 43*, 343-354.

Harris, T., Cook, D. G., Victor, C., DeWilde, S., and Beighton, C. (2006). Onset and persistence of depression in older people: Results from a 2-year community follow-up study. *Age and Ageing, 25*, 25-32.

Hasher, L., and Zacks, R. T. (1988). Working memory, comprehension, and aging: A review and a new view. In G. H. Bower (Ed.), *The psychology of learning and motivation* (Vol. 22, pp. 193-225). New York: Academic Press.

Hershey, D. A., Jacobs-Lawson, J. M., Walsh, D. A. (2003). Influences of age and training on script development. *Aging, Neuropsychology, and Cognition, 10*(1), 1-19.

Houts, P. S., Doak, C. C., Doak, L. G., and Loscalzo, M. J. (2006). The role of pictures in improving health communication: A review of research on attention, comprehension, recall, and adherence. *Patient Education and Counseling, 61*, 173-190.

Houts, P. S., Witmer, J. T., Egeth, H. E., Loscalzo, M. J., and Zabora, J. R. (2001). Using pictographs to enchance recall of spoken medical instructions II. *Patient Education and Counseling, 43*(3), 231-242.

Howard, D. H., Gazmararian, J., and Parker, R. M. (2005). The impact of low health literacy on the medical costs of Medicare managed care enrollees. *The American Journal of Medicine, 118*(4), 371-377.

Institute of Medicine (2004). *Health Literacy: A Prescription to End Confusion.* Washington, D.C.: National Academy of Sciences Press.

Isaacowitz, D. M., Loeckenhoff, C., Wright, R., Sechrest, L., Riedel, R., Lane, R. A., et al. (2007). Age differences in recognition of emotion in lexical stimuli and facial expressions. *Psychology and Aging, 22*, 147-159

Jacobson, T. A., Thomas, D. M., Morton, F. J., Offutt, G., Shevlin, J., and Ray, S. (1999). Use of low-literacy patient education tool to enhance pneumococcal vaccination rates: A randomized controlled trial. *Journal of American Medical Association, 282*(7), 646-650.

Jacoby, L. L., Jennings, J. M., and Hay, J. F. (1996). Dissociating automatic and consciously controlled processes: Implication for diagnosis and rehabilitation of memory deficits. In D. J. Herrmann, C. L. McEvoy, C. Hertzog, P. Hertel, and M. K. Johnson (Eds.), *Basic and applied memory research: Vol. 1. Theory in context* (pp. 161-193). Mahwah, NJ: Erlbaum.

Johnson, M.M.S. (1990). Age differences in decision making: A process methodology for examining strategic information processing. *Journal of Gerontology, 45,* P75-P78.

Johnson, M. M. S., and Drungle, S. C. (2000). Purchasing over-the-counter medications: The impact of age differences in information processing. *Experimental Aging Research*, 26, 245-261.

Kaplan, S. H., Gandek, B., Greenfield, S., Rogers, W., and Ware, J. E. (1995). Patient and visit characteristics related to physicians' participatory decision-making style. *Medical Care, 33*(12), 1176–1187.

Kaufman, D. W., Kelly, J. P., Rosenberg, L., Anderson, T. E., and Mitchell, A. A. (2002). Recent patterns of medication use in the ambulatory adult population of the United States. *Journal of American Medical Association, 287*(3), 337-344.

Kliegel, M., and Martin, M. (2007). Adult age difference in errand planning: The role of task familiarity and cognitive resources. *Experimental Aging Research, 33*, 145-161.

Kline, D. W., and Schreiber, F. (1985). Vision and aging. In J. E. Birren and K. W. Schaie (Eds) *Handbook of the Psychology of aging* (2nd Ed.). New York: Van Nostrand Reinhold.

Kline, D. W. (1994). Optimizing the visibility of displays for older observers. *Experimental Aging Research, 20*(1), 11-23.

Kools, M., van de Wiel, M. W. J., Ruiter, R. A. C., and Kok, G. (2006). Pictures and text in instructions for medical devices: Effects on recall and actual performance. *Patient Education and Counseling, 64*(1-3), 104-111.

Koo, M., Krass, L., and Aslani, P. (2006). Enhancing patient education about medicines: Factors influencing reading and seeking of written medicine information. *Health Expectations, 9*, 174-187.

Kreps, G. L., and Sparks, L. (2008). Meeting the health literacy needs of immigrant populations. *Patient Education and Counseling, 71(3),* 328-332.

Kressig, R. W., and Echt, K. V. (2002). Exercise prescribing: Computer application in older adults. *The Gerontological Society of American, 42*, 273-277.

Kripalani, S., Robertson, R., Love-Ghaffari, M. H., Henderson, L. E., Praska, J., Strawder, A., et al. (2007). Development of an illustrated medication schedule as a low-literacy patient education tool. *Patient Education and Counseling, 66*(3), 368-377.

Kutner, M., Greenberg, E., Jin, Y., Paulsen, C. (2006). *The Health Literacy of America's Adults: Results from the 2003 National Assessment of Adult Literacy* (NCES 2006-483). Washington, DC: National Center for Education Statistics, US Department of Education.

Lea, R. B., and Mulligan, E. J. (2002). The effect of negation on deductive inferences. *Journal of Experimental Psychology: Learning, Memory, and Cognition, 28*, 303-317.

LeDoux, J. (1996). *The emotional brain.* New York: Simon and Schuster.

Lerner, J. S., and Keltner, D. (2000). Beyond valence: Toward a model of emotion-specific influences on judgment and choice. *Cognition and Emotion, 14*, 473-494.

Lerner, J. S., and Keltner, D. (2001). Fear, anger, and risk. *Journal of Personality and Social Psychology, 81*(1), 146-159.

Lerner, J. S., Gonzalez, R. M., Small, D. A., and Fischhoff, B. (2003). Effects of fear and anger on perceived risks of terrorism: A national field experiment. *Psychological Science, 14*, 144-150.

Leventhal, H., Diefenbach, M. A., and Leventhal, E. A. (1992). Illness cognition: Using common sense to understand treatment adherence and affect cognition interactions. *Cognitive Therapy and Research, 16*, 142-163.

Levinson, W., Kao, A., Kuby, A., Thisted, R. A. (2005). Not all patients want to participate in decision making: A national study of public preferences. *Journal of General Internal Medicine, 20*(6), 531-535.

Lewis, D. K., Robinson, J., and Wilkinson, E. (2003). Factors involved in deciding to start preventive treatment: Qualitative study of clinicians' and lay people's attitudes. *British Medical Journal, 327*(7419), 841-846.

Liu, L. L., and Park, D. C. (2004). Aging and medical adherence: The use of automatic processes to achieve effortful things. *Psychology and Aging, 19*(2), 318-325.

Loewenstein, G. F., Hsee, C. K., Weber, E. U., and Welch, N. (2001). Risk as feelings. *Psychological Bulletin, 127*(2), 267-286.

Loewenstein, G. and Lerner, J. (2003). The role of emotion in decision making. In. R.J. Davidson, H. H. Goldsmith, and K. R. Scherer, *Handbook of Affective Science*. Oxford, England: Oxford University Press.

MacDonald, M. C., and Just, M. A. (1989). Changes in activation level with negation. *Journal of Experimental Psychology: Learning, Memory, and Cognition, 15*, 633-642.

MacLaughlin, E. J., Raehl, C. L., Treadway, A. K., Sterling, T. L., Zoller, D. P., and Bond, C. A. (2005). Assessing medication adherence in the elderly? Which tools to use in clinical practice? *Drugs and Aging, 22*(3), 231-255.

Mandelblatt, J., Kreling, B., Figeuriedo, M., and Feng, S. (2006). What is the impact of shared decision making on treatment and outcomes for older women with breast cancer? *Journal of Clinical Oncology: Official Journal of the American Society of Clinical Oncology, 24*(30), 4908-4913.

Maner, J. K., and Schmidt, N. B. (2006). The role of risk avoidance in anxiety. *Behavior Therapy, 37*(2), 181-189.

Mata, R., Schooler, L. J., and Rieskamp, J. (2007). The aging decision maker: Cognitive aging and the adaptive selection of decision strategies. *Psychology and Aging, 22*(4), 796-810.

Mather, M., and Carstensen, L. L. (2003). Aging and attentional biases for emotional faces. *Psychological Sciences, 14*, 409-415.

Mayeaux, E. J., Jr., Murphy, P. W., Arnold, C., Davis, T. C., Jackson, R. H., and Sentell, T. (1996). Improving patient education for patients with low literacy skills. *American Family Physician*, 53(1), 205-211.

Meltzer M. (2008). The mystery of increased hospitalizations of elderly patients. *Emerging Infectious Diseases, 14*(5), 847-848.

Meyer, B. J., Russo, C., and Talbot, A. (1995). Discourse comprehension and problem solving: Decisions about the treatment of breast cancer by women across the life span. *Psychology and Aging, 10*(1), 84-103.

Mireles, D. E., and Charness, N. (2002). Computational explorations of the influence of structured knowledge on age-related cognitive decline. *Psychology and Aging, 17*(2), 245-259.

Morrell, R. W., Park, D. C., Poon, L. W. (1989). Quality of instructions on prescription drug labels: Effects on memory and comprehension in young and old adults. *The Gerontologist, 29*, 345-354.

Morrow, D., and Leirer, V. O., (1999). Designing medication instructions for older adults. In D. C. Park, R. W. Morrell, and K. Shifren (Eds.), *Processing of medical information in aging patients* (pp. 249–265). Mahwah, NJ: Erlbaum.

Morrow, D. G., Leirer, V. O., Andrassy, J. M., Hier, C. M., and Menard, W. E. (1998). The influence of list format and category headers on age differences in understanding medication instructions. *Experimental Aging Research, 24*(3), 231-256.

Moser, R. P., McCaul, K., Peters, E., Nelson, W., and Marcus, S. E. (2007). Associations of perceived risk and worry with cancer health-protective actions: Data from the Health Information National Trends Survey (HINTS). *Journal of Health Psychology, 12*(1), 53-65.

Mroczek, D. K., and Almeida, D. M. (2004). The effect of daily stress, personality, and age on daily negative affect. *Journal of Personality, 72*(2), 354-378.

Naik, A. D., Kallen, M. A., Walder, A., and Street, R. L., Jr. (2008). Improving hypertension control in diabetes mellitus: The effects of collaborative and proactive health communication. *Circulation, 117*(11), 1361-1368.

National Center for Health Statistics. (2003). *Aging boomers drive up doctor visits: Diagnostic tests and prescriptions also on increase*. Washington, DC: Author. Retrieved November 30, 2008, from http://www.cdc.gov/od/oc/media/pressrel/r030811.htm

National Institute on Deafness and other Communications Disorders. (2001). *Hearing loss and older adults* (National Institute of Aging Publication No. 01-4913). Bethesda, MD: NIDCD Information Clearinghouse.

Nielsen-Bohlman, L., Panzer, A. M., and Kindig, D. A. (Eds.). (2004). *Health literacy: A prescription to end confusion*. Washington, D. C.: National Academies Press.

Nisbett, R., and Ross, L. (1980). *Human inference: Strategies and short-comings of social judgment*. Englewood Cliffs, NJ: Prentice Hall.

Nothwehr, F., and Yang, J. (2007). Goal setting frequency and the use of behavioral strategies related to diet and physical activity. *Health Education Research, 22*(4), 532-538.

Nussbaum, J. F., Pecchioni, L., Robinson, J. D., and Thompson, T. (2000). *Communication and aging* (2nd ed.). Mahwah, NJ: Erlbaum.

O'Hara, R., Brooks, J. O., III, Friedman, L., Schröder, C. M., Morgan, K. S., and Kraemer, H. C. (2007). Long-term effects of mnemonic training in community-dwelling older adults. *Journal of Psychiatric Research, 41*(7), 585-590.

O'Hair, H. D.. and Sparks, L. (2008) Relational agency in life threatening illnesses. In K.Wright and S.D. Moore (Eds), *Applied health communication* (pp. 271-289) Creskill, NJ: Hampton Press.

Paasche-Orlow, M. K., Schillinger, D., Greene, S. M., and Wagner, E. H. (2006). How health care systems can being to address the challenge of limited literacy. *Journal of General Internal Medicine, 21*, 884-887.

Park, D., and Schwarz, N. (Eds.). (2000). *Cognitive aging: A primer*. Philadelphia, PA: Psychology Press.

Park, D. C. (1999). Aging and the controlled and automatic processing of medical information and medical intentions. In D. C. Park, R. W. Morrell, and K. Shifren (Eds.), *Processing of medical information in aging patients: Cognitive and human factors perspectives* (pp. 3–22). Mahwah, NJ: Erlbaum.

Park, D. C., and Hall-Gutchess, A. (2000). Cognitive aging and everyday life. In D. C. Park and N. Schwarz (Eds.), *Cognitive aging: A primer* (pp. 217-232.). Philadelphia, PA: Psychology Press.

Park, D. C., Hertzog, C., Leventhal, H., Morrell, R. W., Leventhal, E., Birtchmore, D., et al. (1999). Medication adherence in rheumatoid arthritis patients: Older is wiser. *Journal of the American Geriatrics Society, 47*, 172-183.

Park, D. C., and Jones, T. R. (1996). Medication adherence and aging. In A. D. Fisk and W. A. Rogers (Eds.), *Handbook of human factors and the older adult* (pp. 257-288). San Diego, CA: Academic Press.

Park, D. C., Morrell, R. W., Frieske, D., and Kincaid, D. (1992). Medication adherence behaviors in older adults: Effects of external cognitive supports. *Psychology and Aging, 7*, 252-256.

Parker, R. (2000). Health literacy: A challenge for American Patients and their health care providers. *Health Promotion International, 15*(4), 277-283.

Peters, E., and Slovic, P. (1996). The role of affect and worldviews as orienting dispositions in the perception and acceptance of nuclear power. *Journal of Applied Social Psychology, 26*, 1427-1453.

Petrisek, A. C., Laliberte, L. L., Allen, S. M., and Mor, V. (1997). The treatment decision-making process: Age differences in a sample of women recently diagnosed with nonrecurrent, early-stage breast cancer. *Gerontologist, 37*(5), 598-608.

Pichora-Fuller, M. K., Schneider, B. A., and Daneman, M. (1995). How young and old adult listen to and remember speech in noise. *The Journal of the Acoustical Society of American, 97*(1), 593-608.

Raghunathan, R., and Pham, M. T. (1999). All negative moods are not equal: Motivational influences of anxiety and sadness on decision making. *Organizational Behavior and Human Decision Processes, 79*, 56-77.

Rabbit, P. (1990). Mild hearing loss can cause apparent memory failures which increase with age and reduce with IQ. *Acta oto-laryngologica. Supplementum, 476*, 167-175.

Ratzan, S. C., Lesar, G. L., and Filerman, J. W. (2000). Attaining global health: Challenges and opportunities. *Population Bulletin of the Population Reference Bureau, 55*(1), 3-48.

Richard, R., de Vries, N. K., and van der Pligt, J. (1998). Anticipated regret and precautionary sexual behavior. *Journal of Applied Social Psychology, 28*(15), 1411-1428.

Rogers, W. A., Rousseau, G. K., and Lamson, N. (1999). Maximizing the effectiveness of the warning process: Understanding the variables that interact with age. In D. C. Park, R. W. Morrell, and K. Shifren (Eds.), *Processing of medical information in aging patients: Cognitive and human factors perspectives* (pp. 267-290). Mahwah, NJ: Erlbaum.

Rudd, R., Kirsch, I., and Yamamoto, K. (2004). *Literacy and health in American.* Princeton, NJ: Educational Testing Service.

Safeer, R. S., and Keenan, J. (2005). Health literacy: The gap between physicians and patients. *The American Family Physician, 72*(3), 463-468.

Salthouse, T. A. (1991). *Theoretical perspectives on cognitive aging.* Hillsdale, NJ: Erlbaum.

Salthouse, T. A. (1992). Reasoning and spatial abilities. In F. I. M. Craik and T. A. Salthouse (Eds.), *The handbook of aging and cognition* (pp. 167-211). Hillsdale, NJ: Erlbaum.

Salthouse, T. A. (2000). Item analyses of age relations on reasoning tests. *Psychology and Aging, 15*(1), 3-8.

Salthouse, T. A., Hambrick, D. Z., Lukas, K. E., and Dell, T. C. (1996). Determinants of adult age differences on synthetic work performance. *Journal of Experimental Psychology: Applied, 2*(4), 305-329.

Sanfey, A. G., and Hastie, R. (2000). Judgment and decision making across the adult life span: A tutorial review of psychological research. In D. C. Park and N. Schwarz (Eds.), *Cognitive aging: A primer* (pp. 253-273). Philadelphia, PA: Psychology Press.

Schneider, B., and Pichora-Fuller, M. K. (2000). Implication of sensory deficits for cognitive aging. In F. I. M. Craik, and T. A. Salthouse (Eds.), *The handbook of aging and cognition* (2nd ed.) (pp. 151-220). Hillsdale, NJ: Erlbaum.

Schulman-Green, D., Naik, A., McCorkle, R., Bradley, E. H. and Bogardus, S. (2005). Goat setting as a shared decision making strategy among clinicians and their older patients. *Patient Education and Counseling, 63*(1), 145-151.

Schwartzberg, J. G., Cowett, A., VanGeest, J., and Wolf, M. S. (2007). Communication techniques for patients with low health literacy: A survey of physicians, nurses, and pharmacists. *American Journal of Health Behavior, 31*(S1), S96-S104.

Shiv, B., and Huber, J. (2000). The impact of anticipating satisfaction on consumer choice. *Journal of Consumer Research, 27*, 202-216.

Shohet, L. and Renaud, L. (2006). Critical analysis on best practices in health literacy. *Canadian Journal of Public Health, 97*(S2), S10-3

Slovic, P., Finucane, M., Peters, E., and MacGregor, D. G. (2002). The affect heuristic. In T. Gilovich, D. Griffin, and D. Kahneman (Eds.), Heuristics and biases (pp. 397-410). New

Sparks, L. and Nussbaum, J. F. (2008). Health literacy and cancer communication with older adults. *Patient Education and Counseling, 71*(3), 345-350.

Sparks, L., and Turner, M. M. (2008). Cognitive and emotional processing of cancer messages and information seeking with older adults. In L. Sparks, H. D. O'Hair, and G. L. Kreps, (Eds.), *Cancer communication and aging* (pp. 17-45). Cresskill, NJ: Hampton Press.

Steginga, S. K., Occhipinti, S., Gardiner, R. A.., Yaxley, J., and Heathcote, P. (2002). Making decisions about treatment for localized prostate cancer. *BJU International, 89*(3), 255-260.

Sudore, R. L., Mehta, K. M., Simonsick, E. M., Harris, T. B., Newman, A. B., Satterfield, S., et al. (2006). Limited literacy in older people and disparities in health and healthcare access. *Journal of American Geriatrics Society, 54*, 770-776.

Sullivan, S., Ruffman, T., and Hutton, S. B. (2007). Age difference in emotion recognition skills and the visual scanning of emotion faces. *The Journals of Gerontology Series B: Psychological Sciences and Social Sciences, 62*, P53-P60.

The American Consumer Institute (2006). *Who use information technology services? A demographic analysis of American consumers*. Author: Reston, VA.

Tun, P. A., O'Kane, G., and Wingfield, A. (2002). Distraction by competing speech in younger and older listeners. *Psychology and Aging, 17,* 453–467

United States Department of Education, Institute of Education Sciences, National Center for Education Statistics (NCES). (2003). *National Assessment of Adult Literacy (NAAL).* Washington, DC: NCES.

United States Department of Health and Human Services. (2000). *Healthy people 2010: With understanding and improving health and objectives for improving health* (2nd ed., Vol. 2). Washington, DC: U.S. Government Printing Office.

van Dijk, S., van Roosmalen, M. S., Otten, W., and Stalmeier, P. F. M. (2008). Decision making regarding prophylactic mastectomy: Stability of preferences and the impact of anticipated feelings of regret. *Journal of Clinical Oncology, 26*(14), 2358-2363.

Walsh, D. A., and Hershey, D. A. (1993). Mental models and the maintenance of complex problem-solving skills in old age. In J. Cerella, J. M. Rybash, W. Hoyer, M. L. Commons (Eds.) *Adult information processing: Limits on loss* (pp. 553-584). San Diego, CA: Academic Press.

Weinstein, N. D. (1989). Effects of personal experience on self-protective behavior. *Psychological Bulletin, 105*(1), 31-50.

White, S. (2008). *Assessing the nation's health literacy: Key concepts and findings of the national assessment of adult literacy (NAAL*). Washington, DC: American Medical Association Foundation.

Williams, M. V., Davis, T., Parker, R. M., and Weiss, B. D. (2002). The role of health literacy in patient-physician communication. *Family Medicine, 34*(5), 383-389.

Wilson, E. A. H., and Park, D. C. (2008). A case for clarity in the writing of health statements. *Patient Education and Counseling, 72*, 330-335.

Wingfield, A. (2000). Speech perception and the comprehension of spoken language in adult aging. In D. C. Park and N. Schwarz (Eds.), *Cognitive aging: A primer* (pp. 175-195). Philadelphia, PA: Psychology Press.

Wolf, M. S., Gazmararian, J. A, and Baker, D. W. (2005). Health literacy and functional health status among older adults. *Archives of Internal Medicine, 165*, 1946-1952.

Wolf, M. S., Williams, M. V., Parker, R. M., Parikh, N. S., Nowlan, A. W., and Baker, D. W. (2007). Patients' shame and attitudes toward discussing the results of literacy screening. *Journal of Health Communication, 12*(8), 721-732.

Wood, S., Busemeyer, J., Koling, A., Cox, C. R., and Davis, H. (2005). Older adults as adaptive decision makers: Evidence from the Iowa gambling task. *Psychology and Aging, 20,* 220–225.

Wright, K. B., Sparks, L., and O'Hair, H. D. (2007). *Health communication in the 21st century.* Oxford, England: Blackwell.

Zacks, R. T., Hasher, L., and Li, K. Z. H. (2000). Aging and memory. In T. A. Salthouse and F. I. M. Craik (Eds.), *Handbook of aging and cognition* (pp. 293-357). Hillsdale, NJ: Erlbaum.

Zautra, A. J., Affleck, G. G., Tennen, H., Reich, J. W., and Davis, M. C. (2005). Dynamic approaches to emotions and stress in everyday life: Bolger and Zuckerman reloaded with positive as well as negative affects. *Journal of Personality, 73*, 1511-1538.

Zwahr, M. D., Park, D. C., Eaton, T. A., and Larson, E. (1997). Implementation of the Patient Self-Determination Act: A comparison of nursing homes to hospital. *Journal of Applied Gerontology, 16*, 190-207.

In: New Directions in Aging Research
Editor: Ruby R. Brougham, pp. 119-144
ISBN 978-1-60741-976-1
© 2009 Nova Science Publishers, Inc.

Chapter 7

Age Differences in Response to Time Pressures on Information Processing During Decision Making

***Mitzi Schumacher**[*1] **and Joy M. Jacobs-Lawson**[2]*
[1]College of Medicine, University of Kentucky, Lexington, Kentucky, USA
[2]University of Kentucky, Lexington, Kentucky, USA

Abstract

In the aging literature, it is well established that a number of basic cognitive abilities, including information processing speed, decline with age. It is also known that older adults often develop strategies to adapt to these changes. Although the literature in decision making has examined the effect of age on decision outcomes, less research has focused on age differences in decision processes. This chapter reports on the findings from two studies that examined how older adults use adaptive strategies to make real-world decisions under time constraints. In Study 1, total time for decision processing was limited. Results showed that younger and older adults used different strategies but made similar decisions. In the second study, the time for viewing each piece of information was fixed rather than self-paced. Results showed that the adaptation of the young, but not older adults, resulted in different decisions — indicative of lowering their decision criteria. Consistent with Study 1, older adults increased their organization of information searches. Finally, differences in subsequent mood and metacognitive beliefs in Study 2 suggested differential effects for the experimental manipulations used in Studies 1 and 2. Together, these studies suggest that older adults' information processing strategies are influenced by time pressures.

* Address correspondence to Mitzi Schumacher, Behavioral Science Department, University of Kentucky Medical Center, Lexington KY 40536-0086; E-mail: mitzi.schumacher@uky.edu

Introduction

It is well accepted that aging is associated with a decline in primary mental functions, such as the rate of information processing in learning, memory or visual-spatial tasks. Typically, in the cognitive literature, it is reported that younger participants outperform older adults on those basic functions. However, this is not always the case. This is particularly true when examining higher order cognitive functions such as decision making and when examining the outcomes of individuals decisions. The present chapter presents two studies that focus on the effects of age and time pressure on information processing as individuals make a real-world decision. The chapter is organized as follows: (a) theories of cognitive aging and decision making, (b) research on information processing and aging, (c) Study 1, (d) Study 2, and (e) general discussion.

Relevant Theories of Cognitive Aging and Decision Making

Several theories have emerged to account for age differences in higher order cognitive functioning, such as decision making. The theories that are most relevant to the present study are those concerning: (a) speed of processing (Salthouse, 1991), (b) selection, optimization, and compensation (Baltes and Baltes, 1990), and (c) cognitive potential (Perlmutter, 1988). The cognitive slowing theory argues that any age differences in decision making are due to age-related declines in information processing skills and abilities, which interfere with individuals' ability to select, manipulate and combine information to reach a decision. In contrasts, compensation may play a critical role in older adults' abilities to process information given the declines that exist in the basic skills needed to make decisions (e.g. attention, see McDowd and Shaw, 2000), information processing (Salthouse 2000), and executive functioning (Friedman, Nessler, Johnson, Ritter, and Bersick, 2008). Cognitive potential argues that in light of the declines, strategies are associated with higher order functioning. In order to overcome these declines, older adults may develop strategies or heuristics that they use as decision aids. Consistent with the selection optimization compensation theory in that it could be argued that knowledge and higher mental functions help to compensate for declines in basic cognitive abilities. Perlmutter speculated that the overlay of higher mental functions and world knowledge upon primary mental functions allows older adults to effectively perform despite minor perturbations in primary mental functions.

The notion that older adults use strategies to compensate for declines in basic cognitive abilities is consistent with bounded rationality (Gigerenzer and Selten, 1999) which maintains that in most cases individuals do not consider all information available but rather use heuristics when making decisions. Heuristics are strategies that serve to reduce the cognitive demands of the decision making processes – strategies that are likely to be used by individuals who have fewer cognitive resources, such as older adults, those making complex decisions that require consideration of a large amount of data, those making decisions under duress, or those under time pressures, as in the case of the present study. Examples of heuristics include using recommendations from others, and eliminating options based on the attributes most important to you, and satisficing (i.e. looking for an alternative which is 'good enough' to satisfy minimal decision criteria)(Payne, Bettman and Johnson, 1993; Simon, 1955; 1967). These types of strategies are considered noncompensatory because rather than evaluating all available information, the decision maker only considers a subset of the information.

Information Processing, Decision Making, and Aging

The following section reviews the literature pertaining to cognitive aging and decision making. It begins with a discussion of the literature on information processing and ends with a presentation of the literature on aging and decision making.

Aging and information processing. Perhaps the most well-established empirical finding in cognitive aging is the difference in information processing rates of younger and older adults. This finding has been replicated across a wide variety of cognitive tasks and spans over 50 years of experimental work. For example, early work in the rate of presentation for paired associate learning reported age differences in learning (Korchin and Basowitz, 1957). Later work in memory scanning found that older adults scan items in memory at a slower rate than younger adults, about 14 compared to 26 items per second (Anders, Fozord, and Lillyquist, 1972). Cerella (1990) summarizing these findings, reported that the ratios comparing rates of slowing for basic cognitive processes of younger and older adults are 1.25-1.35 for perceptual processes and 1.8-2.0 for memory scanning and mental rotation. Furthermore, recent studies have confirmed that speed of processing declines with age (Salthouse 2000; Sheppard and Vernon, 2008).

Recent studies suggest that these declines may be reduced through training or participation in engaged activities with others (Stine-Morrow, Parisi, Morrow and Park, 2008; Tranter and Koutstaal, 2008; Willis, et al., 2006). Others have proposed that experience, knowledge, or training in a given area can serve as a buffer and reduce the effects that these declines have on higher level processing (Charness, Kelley, Bosman, and Mottram, 2001; Hershey, Jacobs-Lawson, and Walsh, 2003; Salthouse 1984).

Information processing speed, theoretically considered as a cognitive resource, is often offered as an explanation for findings of age-associated differences in cognitive performance. Salthouse (1991) pointed out there is widespread agreement that "the more rapid execution of cognitive operations allows more, and possibly better, processing to be carried out." Age-associated slowing of basic cognitive processes may limit the amount of information that can be processed in a fixed amount of time or it may affect the depth or completeness of processing; older adults may require more time to process the same amount of information. Thus, problem solutions, information processing, plans or the outcomes of decision making may be compromised by information processing rate requirements.

Research on Decision Making and Aging

Research on aging and decision making grew out of findings from the problem solving literature. The early problem solving literature which used tasks such as "20 questions" clearly showed that problem solving abilities declined with age (Hartley and Anderson, 1983; Denney 1985). However, these works were criticized due to a lack of realism. Denney, et al. (1989; 1992) were among the first to begin examining age differences in real-world problem solving. Consistent with these earlier works, more recent studies of problem solving and aging have demonstrated age-related changes in everyday problem solving performance (Allaire and Marsiske, 2002). One criticism of many of these studies was that they tend to focus on outcome and not the actual process that individuals use to reach their decisions.

Most of the studies that have focused on the *how* of decision making have examined age differences in decision time and amount of information considered. With respect to time, some studies have failed to find age differences in the overall amount of time needed to make a decision in various domains. For example, studies of decisions regarding insurance (Hartley, 1990), retirement plans (Hershey, Walsh, Read, and Chulef, 1990), car buying (Johnson, 1990), apartment rental (Johnson, 1993), and over the counter medication selection (Johnson and Drungle, 2000) failed to show that older adults need more time to make the decision. Other works revealed age-related differences in total time to decision regarding apartments (Johnson, 1997) and political candidates (Riggle and Johnson, 1996). In contrast, the most reliable finding across decision studies involving cars, apartments, and political candidates is the difference in the average time (in seconds) spent viewing individual pieces of information while gathering sufficient information to make a final decision. Consistent with this, several studies have shown that older adults spend from one and a half to two times longer than younger adults viewing individual pieces of information (Johnson, 1990; 1993; 1997; Riggle and Johnson, 1996). Thus, it would seem that there is slowing during information processing which sometimes, but not always, results in a longer time to make the decision.

Time, however, is only one index measuring decision making performance; other indices include information use, organization of information searches, as well as decision outcomes. Studies that have focused on the organization of information have shown that older and younger adults differ in how they process information. In fact, Hershey, Jacobs-Lawson, and Walsh (2003) found training and age influence information processing when making a series of complex decisions. A study of over the counter medication decision have found that older adults were more organized in their information searches but were slower to review information than younger adults (Johnson and Drungle, 2000). Johnson and Ryan (2003) found that when information was presented in an organized fashion, participants were more organized in how they reviewed the information. Such findings indicate that there may also be age differences in the strategies used to make decisions.

Neither time to decision nor time spent viewing information has been consistently linked to these other indices. For example, age differences in decision times were not related to decision outcomes as none of the above studies reported any age-related differences in decision outcomes (Hartley, 1990; Hershey, et al., 1990; Johnson, 1990; 1993;1997; Riggle and Johnson, 1996). However, these studies allowed participants to view information and to make decisions at their own pace. It is not clear whether decision-making performance would suffer if either decision completion time or time allowed to process information was limited. In the literature, time pressure has been shown to influence young adults' decision strategies and information search and decision (Edland, 1994; Maule, Hockey, and Bdzola, 2000). Furthermore, it is not clear how time pressure will modify individuals' memory of the information associated with the decision or how measures of cognitive functioning will be related to information processing under time constraints. Although recent studies have begun to examine the links between cognitive abilities and everyday problem solving (Allaire and Marsiske, 2002; Burton, Strauss, Hultsch, and Hunter, 2006), it is not clear the how they influence information processing in decision making.

The goal of the present inquiry was to examine age differences in the primary and higher mental functioning of younger and older adults by manipulating the time available for completion of decision processes (Study 1) and the time available for viewing information (Study 2). These manipulations should affect the decision performance of younger and older adults differently due to the age-related slowing of information processing. More specifically based on the theories and research discussed above we anticipate that if older, compared to younger adults, compensate for their slower rates of information when time is limited, then they should employ decision rules and information search strategies that require less information and are highly organized and selective. At the same time, they will still have a poorer memory of the information due to age-related decrements in primary mental functions. In contrast, if older adults are simply at a disadvantage, compared to young adults, due to their slower information processing, then when time is limited they will use less information in a less organized way which may result in different decision outcomes as well as poorer memory for information that was inadequately processed in order to make their decision. The findings from the study will have implications for future studies examining the role of stress on the decision making process.

Study 1: Limiting Time to Decision

Maule and Svenson (1993) summarized the findings of the experimental manipulation of time, stating that time constraints lead to less information being processed, greater selectivity of information, faster processing, and in some cases more feature-based searches of the available information. Feature-based searches are those in which features, like price or color, are compared across all alternatives, instead of reviewing all the information about each of the alternatives. Edland and Svenson (1993) further delineated some of the effects of time constraints on strategy use, stating that there is an increased use of noncompensatory decision rules which also involves an increased tendency to lock onto one strategy and a decreased openness to alternatives. Noncompensatory strategies are those in which not all of the information is reviewed for each of the alternatives before they are eliminated from further consideration. Theoretical interpretations of these findings emphasize the effect of time on determining resource allocation and inducing affective states. In determining resource allocation, time affects the framing of problems; individuals may use a cost/benefit analysis of strategy use and resources. Time-induced affective states are also associated with cognitive resources in that monitoring the time available for information processing requires resources and increased arousal.

Imposing limits on total time to decision in the present study led to predictions that young adults in the experimental condition with more severe time constraints would engage in faster processing and use less information. Also, young adults would use more feature (as opposed to alternative) based information searches, and show more variation in the information searched across alternatives due to the use of noncompensatory decision rules, in comparison to their peers in the unconstrained time condition. In contrast, older adults would not be able to engage in faster processing due to their decline in basic cognitive abilities. However, older adults would be more organized in their information searches due the use of heuristics or strategic information search patterns. It is possible that decision outcomes would differ between the constrained and unconstrained time conditions if young and older adults lowered their decision criteria. Finally, it is anticipated that in the time constrained condition, older adults' memory for decision-relevant information would be poorer than younger adults'.

Methods

Design Overview

Because the cognitive slowing of older adults posed a confounding factor, time constraints were defined relative to younger and older adults' samples. Data from an earlier study (Johnson, 1997) with identical stimulus materials and task instructions provided the upper and lower quartiles of the time required for a decision for young (350 and 650 seconds) and older adults (600 and 1200 seconds). The lower quartile represented a shortened time and the upper quartile represented an adequate time for most participants to complete their decision-making processes. Setting these limits constituted target times for task completion — not absolute limits; participants were allowed to complete their decision processes after the time expired. A 2 (young versus older adults) by 2 (short versus long time period) experimental design yielded data from explicit information search protocols for a multi-choice, multi-feature decision task.

Participants

Forty-two young adults (M_{age}= 21.5, SD= 3.21) and 40 older adults (M_{age}= 71.6, SD= 6.29) were recruited and paid $10 for their participation. Young adults were recruited from undergraduate psychology and nursing courses at the University of Kentucky. Older adults were recruited from the University of Kentucky Sanders-Brown Center on Aging volunteer subject pool. Samples were compared on measures of age, gender, educational attainment, socio-economic status, health, the Shipley Institute of Living Scale (Shipley, 1967), the Positive and Negative Affect Scale (Lawton, Kleban, Dean, Rajagopal, and Parmelee, 1992), the Need for Cognition Scale (Cacioppo, Petty, and Kao, 1984) and four metamemory subscales focusing on everyday memory, spatial abilities and concentration (Crook and Larrabee, 1992).

Table 1. Means and Standard Deviations for Measures Describing Samples in Study 1

Measures	Young Adults		Older Adults	
	350 sec.	650 sec.	600 sec.	1200 sec.
	N = 22	N =20	N = 20	N = 20
Education (years)	14.9 (.72)	15.0 (1.61)	14.2 (2.13)	14.6 (2.39)
Vocabulary (40 words)	29.1 (3.98)	28.1 (5.14)	32.7 (6.45)	31.6 (5.02)
Abstraction (20 items)	16.3 (2.20)	16.1 (1.78)	10.4 (5.60)	9.2 (4.12)
Positive Affect (5 pts)	1.7 (.33)	1.8 (.39)	1.9 (.30)	1.9 (.35)
Negative Affect (5 pts)	1.1 (.49)	1.0 (.41)	.72 (.25)	.63 (.23)
Need for Cognition (5 pts)	3.7 (.55)	3.7 (.53)	3.5 (.61)	3.5 (.45)
Everyday Memory (5pts)	3.8 (.66)	3.7 (.69)	3.9 (.71)	4.0 (.66)
Spatial Memory (5 pts)	3.8 (.89)	4.1 (.63)	3.4 (.95)	4.2 (.62)
Concent Problems (5 pts)	2.6 (.59)	2.4 (.59)	2.5 (.67)	2.5 (.46)
Frequency of Everday Problems (5 pts)	2.3 (.49)	2.3 (.62)	2.9 (.65)	2.5 (.67)

Table 1 contains the means and standard deviations for measures describing the young and older adults' samples. Some of these descriptive data were not retrievable from the computer program for four young adults (two in each experimental condition). Two (age group) by two (experimental condition) ANOVAs were conducted on all measures. There were no significant main effects for experimental condition or interactions; however, there were several main effects for age group. Older adults compared to younger adults had significantly more positive affect ($F(1, 74)=4.85$, $p<.05$) and less negative affect ($F(1, 74)=21.35$, $p<.01$). Older adults had higher vocabulary skills ($F(1, 74)=8.96$, $p<.01$), but poorer abstract pattern completion skills ($F(1, 74)=55.90$, $p<.01$). Finally, older adults reported that they perceived more frequent everyday memory problems than younger adults ($F(1, 74)=6.31$, $p<.05$).

Procedure

Each subject participated individually in a single experimental session with a laptop computer. Participants received an oral overview and demonstration of the decision task so that they could become familiar with the use of the computer for the task. Then they completed the decision task, a filler task, the recall and recognition tests, a demographic questionnaire, vocabulary and abstraction tests, and self-report measures.

The decision task involved indicating a preference to rent one apartment from among eight. Preference for any apartment represented the "correct" answer. Information was organized in an eight by eight matrix with numbers for the apartments labeling the columns and features (cost, management, floor/decor, appliances, sq. footage, parking, location, and neighbors) labeling the rows. To select a piece of information participants pressed the cursor keys to highlight a cell of the matrix and pressed the "enter" key. Information remained on the screen until participants exited the cell, at which time the cell was marked with an asterisk. At any time during the task, participants could choose an apartment, or re-read the introductory description of the task and instructions regarding how to use the computer. Participants could also choose to display cues for all the information cells they had already viewed (marked with asterisks). This review took the form of a computerized note pad -- to help participants remember information they had previously accessed one piece at a time by showing cues for all the information at the same time. The cues took the form of five character words or abbreviations designed to capture the essence of information contained in each cell of the matrix. Only cells that had been previously accessed revealed cues denoting the information from the cells.

A research assistant instructed participants to complete their deliberations in the time specified in the upper left corner of the computer screen; she stated that this time was the average time required by other participants to make the same decision. The digital clock counted down to the specified time and a tone sounded every 30 seconds. The research assistant also emphasized the importance of time by using a stop watch to monitor participants' progress. Although the research assistant did not stop participants at the end of the time period, she encouraged them to complete the task as quickly as possible.

After a filler task, participants wrote down all the information they could remember about the apartment they had chosen to rent. This was followed by a computerized recognition test in which the decision matrix was displayed again. Individual cells of information randomly appeared and participants were required to decide whether that was the correct information from the decision task. Only cells that the subject had previously accessed were included and half of these displayed information that was incorrect. Both memory tests were self-paced.

Finally, demographic questions, the vocabulary and abstraction tests, and self-report measures were administered by the computer.

Measurement

Cognitive functioning. The Shipley Institute of Living Scale, Positive and Negative Affect Scale, and Need for Cognition Scale served as measures of cognitive functioning in Study 1. The Shipley Institute of Living Scale (Shipley, 1967) consists of forty multiple-choice vocabulary items (serves a measure of knowledge) and twenty series completion problems which required completion of patterns of letters, numbers or words (serves as a indicator of fluid abilities). Scores range from zero to forty for the vocabulary subscale and from zero to twenty for the abstraction subscale. The Positive and Negative Affect Scale (Lawton, et al., 1992) is comprised of five positive and five negative adjective descriptors of affective states. Participants recorded a number from 1 to 5 to describe the extent to which they feel that way at the present time. The Need for Cognition Scale (Cacioppo, Petty and Kao, 1984) contains 16 statements for which participants rated the extent to which the statement described them on a 5-point scale anchored with the phrases "extremely uncharacteristic of me" and "extremely characteristic of me." Finally, four subscales of the

Crook and Larrabee (1992) metamemory scale were included to examine participants' perceptions of their memory. Seven items assessing ability, specifically everyday task-oriented (4 items) and spatial memory (3 items) abilities, were accompanied by a 5-point scale anchored by "very poor" and "very good." Nine items assessing the frequency of problems, specifically attention/concentration (5 items) and everyday task-oriented problems (4 items), were similarly accompanied by a 5-point scale anchored by "very rarely" and "very often."

Decision-making performance measures. The primary advantage of using computerized process tracing techniques is to access measurement of the dynamic aspects of decision making. The computer records the on-going sequence of information requests as well as the time spent engaged in each event. From this record several types of measures are derived. Despite encouraging adherence to the time limits, not all participants completed the task within the time specified; thus indices of time included the total *seconds to decision*, measured from the first appearance of the information matrix until participants indicate they were ready to make their decision. This was also used to create an indicator of time relative to condition, which negative scores indicate the participants completed the task before the specified time lapsed, whereas a positive score indicates how much additional time was needed for them to actually reach a decision. A second time measure was the mean number of *seconds viewing information*, calculated from the time spent viewing discrete pieces of information divided by the number of pieces of information accessed. Indices indicative of information use included the number of pieces of *information viewed* (regardless of repetitions), the *proportion of information* from the matrix calculated from the cells accessed divided by the number of matrix cells (64) and, the number of *repetitions* of requests for previously viewed information.

Measures indicative of the use of decision rules had two components: the organization of information searches and the variation or depth of information searched across alternatives. Search organization indices were calculated as the ratios of requests for information from the same apartment (apartment ratio of repetition) or from the same feature (feature ratio of repetition) divided by the information viewed less the number of matrix dimensions (patterned after subjective organization measures of free recall such as Adjusted Ratio of Clustering (ARC), cf. Murphy and Puff, 1982). In a feature-based organizational strategy a subject would go across the rows to access feature information in the decision matrix. In a choice-based organizational strategy a subject would go up and down the columns in the decision matrix to access information about each choice sequentially. These measures were not combined into a single index (see Böckenholt and Hynan, 1994, for justification) but were analyzed together in a mixed analysis of variance. Variation in search was calculated as the standard deviation of the proportion of information accessed across alternatives. (For example, a subject who looked at 2 of 8 cells for the first alternative, 4 of 8 cells for the second and third alternative, 5 of 8 cells for the fourth alternative and 2 of 8 cells for the last alternative would be assigned a variation score of .1677).

Hand-written free recall protocols were coded for the gist of the information participants had accessed during their information searches; so that if participants accessed only six of eight possible cells of information the percentage of recall was scored on that basis. Similarly, the percent of recognition hits were the number of cells correctly identified divided by the number of cells accessed and the percent of false alarms were the number of cells incorrectly identified as being the original decision matrix information divided by the number of cells accessed.

Because the above measures of time, information use, organization and variation of information searches, and memory reflect distinct constructs with differential theoretical predictions stemming from Perlmutter's (1988) theory, all analyses of variance (ANOVA) were conducted separately for each measure (instead of performing a single omnibus multivariate analysis of variance) with conventional alpha levels.

Results

Decision-Making Performance

Means and standard deviations for measures of time, information use, organization and variation of information searches, and memory for decision-relevant information are presented in Table 2. Most data were analyzed using two (age group) by two (experimental condition) between participants ANOVAs. The exceptions to were the organization measures, which were analyzed using two (age group) by two (experimental condition) by two (measure: feature versus apartment) mixed ANOVAs.

Table 2. Means and Standard Deviations for Measures of Decision Making Performance

Measures	Young Adults		Older Adults	
	350 sec. N = 22	650 sec. N =20	600 sec. N = 20	1200 sec. N = 20
Time				
Sec. to Time Limit	-16.6 (119.92)	-203.7 (165.46)	+43.5 (178.26)	-447.3 (285.22)
Sec. Viewing Info	1.9 (.63)	2.5 (1.02)	4.1 (1.71)	6.2 (4.41)
Information Use				
Information Viewed	39.1 (13.70)	56.5 (22.29)	40.2 (17.64)	42.6 (24.17)
Proportion of Info.	.49 (.18)	.69 (.25)	.55 (.24)	.54 (.31)
Information Repetition	7.5 (6.17)	12.1 (10.99)	5.2 (6.25)	8.2 (9.00)
Search Organization				
Feature Based	.48 (.21)	.53 (.25)	.46 (.34)	.43 (.31)
Choice Based	.39 (.21)	.33 (.26)	.47 (.32)	.50 (.24)
Variation in Info Search Across Alternatives	.28 (.11)	.19 (.15)	.22 (.17)	.19 (.14)

Time. Overall 58 (70.7%) of the participants made their decision within the time limit they were given. Ninety percent of the participants working under long time constraints finished on time; whereas only 52.4% of those working under the shorter time did so. Comparison by age groups revealed that 76.2% of the younger participants and 65.0% of the older participants made their decision with the time constraints provided. ANOVAs revealed significant main effects and an interaction for the difference between the allotted time and the time participants actually took to make their decisions. Participants given a longer period of time made their decisions on average in 325.5 fewer seconds than the allotted time. Older adults given 600 seconds for their decision making took 44 seconds longer than the allotted time, while young adults in both conditions and older adults given a longer period completed their decisions in less time than was allotted ($F(1,78)=12.39$, $p<.01$). There were also main effects for age group and condition on the mean time spent viewing information measure. Older adults spent 5.1 seconds viewing information, compared to young adults who spent 2.2 ($F(1,78)=29.99$, $p<.01$). Participants given a shorter period of time to make decisions on average spent 2.9 seconds viewing information compared to the 4.4 seconds spent by participants given a longer period. No other effects were significant.

Information use. There were main effects for experimental condition on the total amount of information viewed ($F(1,78)=5.10$, $p<.05$) and on repetition of information requests ($F(1,78)=4.24$, $p<.05$). These effects showed that there was less information viewed by participants in the short (39.6 pieces) versus longer time periods (49.5 pieces). Participants in short periods also made fewer repeated requests to see already viewed information than participants in longer periods (6.4 compared to 10.1 requests). No other effects reached significance for measures of information use, although the interaction of age group and experimental condition approached significance for the proportion of information used ($F(1,78)=3.76$, $p=.0561$).

Organization and variation of information search. There was a main effect for age group for the organization of information searches ($F(1,76)=8.53$, $p=.01$) such that older adults were more organized than young adults, .47 compared to .43. No other effects were statistically significant for the organization measures. There was a main effect for experimental condition for the variation of information searched across alternatives ($F(1,78)=9.67$, $p=.01$), indicating that participants given shorter time periods had more variable searches across alternatives than participants given longer time periods (mean comparison of .19 versus .26).

Decision outcomes. Chi square analyses of the data regarding participants' choice of apartments revealed no significant effects associated with either age group or experimental condition.

Memory for decision-relevant information. Free recall data from 11 older adults were uncodable, although their recognition data were retrievable. Analyses of the free recall data revealed a significant main effect for age group ($F(1,67)=6.61$, $p=.05$) and an interaction ($F(1,67)=5.02$, $p=.05$). Young adults given a longer period for their decision processing remembered more information about their final choice than young adults given less time and older adults in both conditions.

Analyses of the recognition data confirmed the main effect for age group on the percent of recognition hits ($F(1,78)=16.13$, $p=.01$), but did not reveal any other significant effects. Young adults recognized 40% of the information they reviewed while making their decision, while older adults recognized approximately 31%.

Discussion

Time to decision confirmed that young and older adults adhered to the time limits and were responsive to the time pressure induced by the computer-generated beeps and the research assistant monitoring a stop watch. Consistent with findings from previous studies imposing limits of time on young adults (Maule and Svenson, 1993), manipulation of time constraints during decision making processes lead to faster processing times, even for older adults. Older adults still took longer, indicating slower information processing rates which were consistent with predictions based on declines in processing abilities; but they did "speed up." This was evidenced by the total time to make decisions and by the time spent viewing matrix cells containing information.

The experimental manipulation also affected information use. Consistent with previous research, all participants given shorter time periods used less information than their peers who were allowed longer time periods (Edland and Svenson, 1993); there were no age-related decrements in information use. Analyses of the variation in information searches confirms the findings of analyses of information use; variation increased in the conditions with greater time constraints with no additional effect associated with age. This finding suggests a mechanism by which young and older adults reduced their information requirements, that is, by using noncompensatory decision rules (Edland and Svenson, 1993). In contrast to research reviewed by Edland and Svenson (1993), there were no increases in the use of feature-based information searches associated with the experimental condition or age. However, consistent with predictions based on age differences in compensation and cognitive potential, there was a main effect for age on organization measures (collapsed across feature and apartment-based) but reduced memory. That older adults were more organized than young adults suggests a potential mechanism by which older adults may have increased their processing speeds. This contradicts other studies that have shown younger adults to be more strategic in their information searches (Hershey, et al., 2003). However, in the Hershey study the goal was to examine information processing over a series of trials to see if both younger and older adults developed information processing scripts when solving financial decisions. The present study used a single decision with time pressures. It is possible that the differences are due to the domain examined (IRA vs apartment) or the fact that in Hershey et al. multiple decisions were made.

Although it was possible that the manipulation could have affected participants' decision criteria, there were no differences in decision outcomes associated with age group or experimental condition. Finally, analyses of the recall and recognition data showed typical age-related differences consistent with predictions based on speed of processing, older adults recalled and recognized less, as well as an effect for experimental condition on young adults' memory for information about their final choice.

Clearly, the manipulation of the time allowed for decision making affected the information processing of young and older adults. However, the experimental manipulation not only limited the time available, it also created a potential distraction from the decision task. Participants' decision processes could have been interrupted by the computer beeps or the researcher's obvious monitoring of the stop watch. This could have made it more difficult for the participants to focus on the task or lead to divided attention, which would have reduced attention resources that could be allotted to the decision (McDowd and Shaw, 2000). This hypothetical secondary effect of the experimental manipulation received some empirical support in this study from analyses of the variation of seconds spent viewing information. Two (age group) by two (experimental condition) ANOVAs using the standard deviations associated with the mean time spent viewing information from the matrix (after log linear transformation) as the dependent measure showed both a main effect for age ($F(1,78)=48.73$, $p<.01$) and an interaction ($F(1,78)=3.97$, $p<.05$) indicating older adults in the long condition had the greatest variation of viewing times ($M=11.6$, $SD=9.23$) compared to older adults in the short condition ($M=7.3$, $SD=3.08$) and young adults in the long ($M=4.2$, $SD=1.02$) and short ($M=4.4$, $SD=1.26$) conditions. In the long time period, older adults spent several seconds viewing individual pieces of information; when reminded by the computer-generated beeps and the presence of the research assistant checking a stopwatch, they sped up their viewing rates only to slow down when the sense of urgency passed. These findings may be due to both the time limit and older adults' awareness of the passage of time. Study 2 addressed the effects of limiting time for decision processes without emphasizing the passage of time.

Study 2

In Study 2 participants were not required to monitor the passage of time in order to complete their decision processes within a set time period; however, the computer presented information from the matrix cells for a fixed period of time. Through computerized control of the viewing time, information processing time was limited while eliminating the distraction of the beeping count down clock and the research assistant's monitoring of the passage of time allowed for making a decision. Due to age-related declines in basic cognitive abilities, limits on processing times should have a greater impact on older adults; therefore information viewing times were set so that one condition represents an average viewing time for normal older adults and the other condition represents an average viewing time appropriate to young adults. The comparison condition for older adults was a faster time and the comparison condition for young adults was a slower time.

Predictions based on age-related differences in cognitive abilities were similar to those of Study 1. First, time to decision will be associated with experimental conditions manipulating time and age differences which will reflect differences in basic cognitive abilities. Second, because the total time to decision was not limited, information use should not be affected. But, because older adults may not have enough time to process individual cells of information and the task allowed participants to request the same piece of information repeatedly, it was also expected that such repetitions would be more frequent for older adults with shorter viewing time. Third, participants would be more likely to organize their information searches using features and to search a variable amount of information across alternatives. This prediction followed from expectations based on previous research with young adults (Edland and Svenson, 1993) and theoretical predictions that primary mental functions would be disrupted. Older adults, in particular, would be more organized in their information requests and adhere to decision rules which reduce processing requirements, such as noncompensatory Elimination by Aspect and Satisficing rules. Based on their review of previous research with young adults, Edland and Svenson (1993) also suggest that decision outcomes may vary as a result of the lowering of decision criteria in the face of limits on information processing. As in Study 1, it was expected that age associated differences in memory would be observed.

Method

Design

Similar to the first study, the design was a between participants, two (age group) by two time condition (short versus long periods allowed for viewing information). Findings from an earlier study using the same task established that younger adults averaged 2 seconds compared to older adults who averaged 5 seconds to view each piece of information when making a decision about which apartment to rent (Johnson, 1997). Thus, the time allowed for information processing for the experimental conditions was set at two seconds and five seconds.

Additional measures of processing speed and working memory using the digit-digit and digit-symbol matching tasks (Salthouse, 1992) and the reading span task (Daneman and Carpenter, 1980) were included in order to characterize the samples and confirm predictions based on age differences in basic cognitive abilities. Data collected on education, vocabulary and abstraction skills (Shipley, 1967), perceived memory abilities and frequency of problems (Crook and Larrabee, 1992), and need for cognition (Cacioppo, Petty and Kao, 1984) were similar to Study 1.

Participants

Younger adults were recruited from undergraduate political science courses. Older adults were recruited from the University of Kentucky Sanders-Brown Center on Aging volunteer subject pool. All participants were paid $10 for their participation. Younger and older adults were randomly assigned; there were 29 younger and 26 older adults in the short (2 second) condition, and 30 younger and 26 older adults in the long (5 second) condition. The mean age of the younger adults was 23.6 years (SD=3.59), and for older adults was 71.5 years (SD=6.46). Participants in Study 2 did not participate in Study 1.

Table 3 contains the means and standard deviations for measures characterizing the samples. Preliminary ANOVAs were conducted to examine any main effects for age, assigned condition, or interactions that would indicate participants differed across conditions. (Data were irretrievable for up to six young adults on various measures, thus degrees of freedom for analyses change.)

There were age differences in years of education ($F(1,102)=41.7$, $p<.01$); abstraction skills ($F(1,98)=66.2$, $p<.01$); self-perceived spatial abilities ($F(1,100)=11.2$, $p<.01$); problems in concentration ($F(1,100)=6.67$, $p<.05$); frequency of everyday memory problems ($F(1,100)=16.3$, $p<.01$); need for cognition ($F(1,100)=36.8$, $p<.01$); reading span

($F(1,105)=31.7$, $p<.01$); digit-digit matching ($F(1,97)=31.0$, $p<.01$); digit-symbol matching ($F(1,99)=96.0$, $p<.01$).

Table 3. Means and Standard Deviations for Measures Describing Samples in Study 2

Measures	Young Adults		Older Adults	
	Short 2 sec. N = 29	Long 5 sec. N =30	Short 2 sec. N = 26	Long 5 sec. N = 26
Education (years)	17.5 (2.46)	16.8 (2.34)	13.9 (2.80)	14.0 (2.55)
Vocabulary (40 words)	31.8 (4.07)	31.1 (3.18)	32.1 (4.52)	31.5 (5.32)
Abstraction (20 items)	15.9 (1.90)	16.5 (1.92)	11.0 (4.45)	10.3 (4.58)
Positive Affect (5 pts)	3.3 (.72)	3.4 (.75)	3.2 (.96)	3.9 (.76)
Negative Affect (5 pts)	1.7 (.54)	1.7 (.75)	1.3 (.42)	1.3 (.40)
Need for Cognition (5 pts)	3.7 (.63)	3.7 (.57)	2.8 (.73)	3.0 (.71)
Everyday Memory (5pts)	3.8 (.68)	3.9 (.57)	3.5 (.76)	4.1 (.78)
Spatial Memory (5 pts)	4.1 (.90)	4.3 (.59)	3.5 (.92)	3.7 (1.03)
Concent Problems (5 pts)	2.1 (.66)	2.4 (.67)	2.8 (.61)	2.3 (.58)
Frequency of Everyday Problems (5 pts)	2.2 (.73)	2.2 (.62)	3.0 (.68)	2.5 (.55)

There were also main effects for condition for self-perceived everyday memory abilities ($F(1,100)=6.5$, $p<.05$) and frequency of everyday memory problems ($F(1,100)=4.0$, $p<.05$). Further interactions qualified the findings for self perceived problems in concentration ($F(1,100)=8.5$, $p<.01$) and frequency of everyday memory problems ($F(1,100)=4.0$, $p<.05$). Because the meta-memory questionnaire followed the decision task and memory tests, it is likely that some participants, especially older adults, in the short condition were more sensitive regarding their memory abilities.

Procedure

As in Study 1, participants complete the study individually using a laptop computer. The decision task was identical to that used in the first study, with the exception that the time allowed to make a decision was not limited and in the short condition the information disappeared after two seconds; in the long condition it disappeared after five seconds.

When participants finished the decision task they completed the digit-digit and digit-symbol task (Salthouse, 1992). In this computerized version, the top of the display consisted of a code table with ten pairs of digits (identical) or digit-symbols which remained constant across trials; below the code table a single test item consisting of one pair varied across trials. Instructions to work as quickly as possible required participants to press the / (slash) key when the test item pair matched one of the pairs of the code table and the Z key when they did not (cf. Salthouse, 1992).

After participants completed surprise self-paced recall and recognition tests (identical to those in Study 1), they completed the reading span measure. In this computerized version of the Daneman and Carpenter task (1980) participants read five blocks of sentences in sets of two, three, four, five and six sentences. After each block, participants recalled the last word of each sentence in the block under the restriction that they could not recall the last word of the last sentence first. As participants progressed through each set they recalled two words, three words, four words, five words and six words. If they could not remember all the last words of the sentences in that block they failed that block. After two failed blocks the research assistant assigned them the number of sentences in the last successfully completed block as their reading span score, so that scores ranged from 2 to 6. Finally, the demographic questions, vocabulary and abstraction tests, and self-report measures specified in Study 1 were administered by the computer.

Dependent Measures

All measures of decision making performance were the same as in Study 1, with the addition of an information use measure specifying the frequency with which participants made two consecutive requests to view the same cell of information. This measure was labeled a double-take since it denotes a rapid or surprised second look at something whose significance had not been completely grasped at first.

Results

Decision-Making Performance Measures

Table 4 contains means and standard deviations for performance measures of decision time, information use, and organization and variation of information searches. Unless otherwise specified all analyses were two (age group) by two (condition) factorial analyses of variance.

Time. As expected, time measures reflected the condition to which participants were assigned; however, there was still a main effect indicating an age-related difference for total time to decision ($F(1,107)=10.0$, $p<.01$). As hypothesized, regardless of assigned condition, older adults took longer to make decisions than young adults.

Information use. The measure of information viewed by participants showed a main effect of time ($F(1,107)=6.2$, $p<.05$). Participants having only two seconds viewed more pieces of information. However, there were no significant main effects or interaction for the proportion of information used. Thus, the first finding of differences due to condition in the number of requests for information was likely due to participants repeating requests for information that had already been accessed. A condition main effect for double-takes confirmed this interpretation and showed that participants in the short condition were more likely to do double-takes than participants in the long condition ($F(1,107)=18.2$, $p<.01$). An age group main effect ($F(1,107)=4.9$, $p<.05$) indicated that older adults were more likely to do double-takes than young adults. Finally, information repetitions (nonconsecutive) also revealed a main effect for condition ($F(1, 107)=6.9$, $p<.01$). Both young and older adults in the short condition were more likely to repeat requests for information already seen than participants in the long condition.

Table 4. Means and Standard Deviations (in parentheses) for Measures of Decision Making Performance

Measures	Young Adults		Older Adults	
	2 sec. N = 29	5 sec. N =30	2 sec. N = 26	5 sec. N = 26
Time				
Sec. to Decision	404.0 (244.90)	545.0 (380.15)	601.8 (263.87)	732.1 (368.80
Information Use				
Information Viewed	72.5 (39.03)	60.2 (28.16)	75.6 (44.09)	54.6 (27.91)
Proportion of Info.	.74 (.28)	.73 (.21)	.74 (.31)	.68 (.30)
Double Takes	9.8 (14.50)	1.9 (3.63)	15.3 (13.88)	5.6 (7.73)
	22.8 (24.39)	15.5 (23.94)	28.4 (32.02)	11.3 (12.70)
Information Repetition				
Search Organization				
Feature Based	.53 (.25)	.58 (.27)	.66 (.27)	.45 (.30)
Choice Based	.44 (.26)	.34 (.25)	.44 (.31)	.53 (.33)
Info Search Variation Across Alternatives	.12 (.13)	.17 (.15)	.17 (.18)	.18 (.16)

Organization and variation of information searches. A two (age group) by two (condition) by two (organizational measure) mixed analysis of variance revealed main effects for age ($F(1,107)=9.3$, $p<.01$), condition ($F(1,107)=7.1$, $p<.01$) and organizational measure ($F(1,107)=5.5$, $p<.05$). These main effects were qualified by a three way interaction ($F(1,107)=4.5$, $p<.05$). Overall, main effects indicate that older adults were more organized in their searches and that feature-based strategies were used more than choice-based strategies. The interaction indicates that while young adults tended to favor feature-based organizational strategies, older adults switched strategies depending on the condition. In the two second condition, older adults favored a feature-based strategy, whereas in the five second condition they favored a choice-based strategy. While these findings confirmed those of Study 1 showing main effects for age, the additional effects associated with condition and measure as well as the interaction suggested differential effects associated with this manipulation. There were no significant effects for the measure of variability of information searched across alternatives.

Decision Outcomes

Table 5 shows the final choices of young and older adults by condition. A two by eight Chi square analysis using age group and apartment chosen revealed a significant association between age and the apartments chosen (X^2 (7,n=111)=14.8, $p<.05$).

Table 5.Decision Outcomes: Percent Subjects Choosing each Apartment by Age and Condition in Study Two

	Young Adults		Older Adults	
Choice	2 sec. N=29	5 sec. N=30	2 sec. N=26	5 sec. N=26
Apartment #1	3.5	10	19.2	19.2
Apartment #2	20.7	30	15.4	30.8
Apartment #3	3.5	3.3	-	-
Apartment #4	37.9	3.3	26.9	30.8
Apartment #5	6.9	23.3	7.7	-
Apartment #6	3.5	10	-	-
Apartment #7	20.7	3.3	26.9	11.5
Apartment #8	3.5	16.7	3.9	7.7

Another two by eight Chi square analysis using condition and apartment chosen also revealed a significant association between condition and the apartments chosen (X^2(7,n=111)=14.5, p<.05). To clarify these findings additional chi square analyses were conducted. The first used the apartment chosen and age groups within each condition. These analyses revealed a significant association between age group and apartment chosen in the long condition only (X^2(7,n=56)=19.1, *p*<.01), such that in the long condition older adults were more likely to choose apartment #4 while young adults were more likely to choose #5. Finally, chi square analysis of the apartment chosen and condition within each age group showed a significant association between condition and apartment chosen for young adults only (X^2(7,n=59)=19.9, *p*<.01); older adults did not choose different apartments across conditions, but young adults did. Young adults in the short condition were much more likely to choose apartment #4 than young adults in the long condition. Because the stimuli were identical to those of Study 1, in which there were no differences in decision outcomes, these findings merited further investigation. Two (age) by two (condition) post hoc ANOVAs for each of the types of information viewed (cost, management, floor/decor, appliances, sq. footage, parking, location, and neighbors), showed that participants in the long condition were more likely to request information on appliances (*F*(1,106)=6.2, *p*<.05) and location (*F*(1,106)=14.7, *p*<.01) than participants in the short condition. Thus, in terms of the last hypothesis, older adults did not arrive at different decision outcomes when less time was allowed for information processing (although young adults did), and this may have been due to additional information viewed during the long condition which affected the choices of young adults but did not affect the choices of older adults.

Memory

Table 4 also contains the means and standard deviations for the free recall and recognition measures. Older compared to young adults recalled less of the information about the specific apartment they choose ($F(1,106)=26.4$, $p<.01$). They also recognized fewer target items ($F(1,106)=9.4$, $p<.01$) and had more false alarms ($F(1,106)=7.8$, $p<.01$) than young adults.

Measures of Cognitive Functioning

After partialling out the effect of age, two of the meta-memory subscales, the Shipley vocabulary and abstraction subscales, and participants' years of education were correlated with measures of decision performance and memory for decision-relevant information. Total time to decision was negatively correlated with perceived frequency of problems with everyday memory (r = -.26, $p<.05$). Information viewed and used were related to concentration (information viewed r =.22, $p<.05$) and negatively correlated with perceived frequency of problems with everyday memory (proportion of information used r = -.24, $p<.05$). Choice-based organization of information searches was negatively correlated with abstraction skills (r = -.26, $p<.05$). Memory for decision-relevant information was related to education (r =.26, $p<.05$) and to vocabulary skills (r =.22, $p<.05$). No other partial correlations involving positive or negative affect, need for cognition, digit-digit, digit-symbol or reading span were significant.

Discussion

Findings from this study were largely consistent with those of Study 1. As in Study 1, analyses of time measures replicated earlier studies (Johnson, 1993; 1997). Consistent with predictions derived from age-related declines in basic abilities, older adults took longer to make their decisions in comparison to young adults. Analyses of information use measures showed the effects of time constraint conditions. These differences were mainly due to young and older adults' requests for information that had already been viewed — sometimes in the form of double-takes. Findings from the organization and variation of information search measures suggested that older adults are more strategic – and can compensate to override declines in processing abilities. Decision outcomes differed for young adults across the two experimental conditions but remained the same for older adults. This finding implies that young adults adapt to some decision contexts by changing their decision criteria; whereas older adults adapted the way they accessed information while keeping the criteria the same. This interpretation is underscored by other researchers investigating the decision processes of young adults (Maule and Svenson, 1993; Benson and Beach, 1996). Finally, memory measures revealed typical age-related differences (favoring young adults) but no differences were associated with processing time condition. This suggests that information was fully processed; partial or shallow processing did not lead to additional memory failure.

Participants, and particularly older adults, became aware of the processing difficulties associated with the shorter viewing time, and adjusted how they examined decision relevant information. That education and vocabulary were related to memory of the information viewed and to organization of information searches fits suggests that these may serve as a buffer for age declines in basic abilities. Surprisingly, digit symbol reactions times and reading span scores (basic cognitive abilities) were not related to time to decision. Several explanations could account for these null findings. It could have been due to the direct manipulation of information viewing time which affected time to decision. It also could have been due to measurement inaccuracies, especially in the case of the reading span task on which most participants scored the same. However, correlational analyses of three alternative scoring methods with more variation in scores (including the total words recalled, the number of blocks successfully completed) yielded significant correlations with memory measures but no significant correlations with other decision performance measures. The null findings could also be due to the small effect size of the relationship and the limited samples in this study. Obviously, more research is needed to fully distinguish the validity of these explanations.

Conclusion

Several theories of cognitive aging were examined in the present chapter. Although there is little research, reviews of the decision processes of young adults (Edland and Svenson, 1993; Maule and Svenson, 1993) suggested that young adults' responses to time limits are characterized by: (a) speeding up information processing; (b) using less information; (c) increasing the organization and variation of information searches; and (d) lowering decision criteria. In Study 1, in which the total time available for decision making was limited, young adults sped up their decision processing and decreased information use; older adults decreased their information use and increased their organization of information searches. This shows that both groups developed different heuristics to aid them in making the decision under the time pressure. In Study 2, in which the presentation time for individual pieces of information was limited, young adults lowered their decision criteria; older adults increased the organization of their information searches. Not only were there age-related differences in response to time limits, but these adaptations were also related to the specific experimental manipulation.

These specific experimental manipulations highlight theoretical distinctions between perceptions of time pressure and time limits. Study 1 invoked a sense of time pressure and varied the time allowed to complete decision processes. Study 2 varied limits on the processing of pieces of decision-relevant information without drawing participants' attentions to time pressures. The difference in these two manipulations can be most clearly seen in terms of the impact on participants' self-reported positive and negative affect and metamemory which were completed after finishing the decision task. In Study, 1 there were no significant effects associated with assignment to experimental condition on these measures; in Study 2 there were several. This distinction suggests that in Study 1 in which participants were clearly aware of the time limits they coped directly with those constraints. Young adults sped up their processing times, whereas older adults were more organized in their information searches. In contrast, in Study 2 with no apparent time pressures for making decisions, the fixed pace for the presentation of information cells disrupted decision processes such that young and older adults repeated their requests for information. The adaptations used by young adults in Study 1 were not used by the young adults in Study 2;

however, the adaptations of older adults in Studies 1 and 2 were similar. While the theoretical distinction between these experimental manipulations has been discussed in reviews of research on young adults (Maule and Svenson, 1993), these studies extended this distinction to studies of older adults and provided empirical support for age-related differences in adaption to perceived time pressure and fixed presentation.

A generalized slowing hypothesis would have predicted simply that when time for information processing was limited the decision making performance of older adults would be impaired. Specifically, in comparison to younger adults, older adults would a) be slower to make decisions, b) use less information, and c) arrive at different decision outcomes. This did not happen in the present studies. Although older adults were slower decision makers, under time limits older adults used the same information in more strategic ways to arrive at the same decision outcomes, in Study 1. These findings highlight the adaptive nature of older adults' everyday cognition, and are consistent with other evidence that older adults adapt when confronted with speeded tasks. For example, Salthouse (1984) reported that even though older typists had slower tapping rates and choice reaction times, their overall typing speed was not slower than that of younger adults because older typists looked further ahead in the text while typing.

These studies provide evidence of age-related differences in adaptation to adverse decision contexts. The primary adaptation used by young adults to cope with time pressure in Study 1 was to increase the speed of their information processing. Although older adults lack this ability, they were able to compensate and used a heuristic to help them make the decision. Further, based on the finding of different decision outcomes for young adults in the short and long conditions of Study 2, their adaptations influenced their final decisions. Benson and Beach (1996) found that when young adults sped up their information processing, it led to inconsistent application of decision criteria while screening alternatives. While this effect was eliminated with instructions emphasizing the importance of the task, in the present studies older adults' needed no such instructions.

The two studies suggest that when making complex decisions, older adults have adapted to limitations in information processing limitations. One way that they showed adaptation was refining the search strategy and being more organized when under stress. This contradicts Hershey et al. (2003) who found that over a series of financial problems, older adults without a strong knowledge of the domain did not develop a strategy to process the information. There are several explanations for this difference. First, in Hershey, et al. (2003) participants requested what information they thought they would need to make the decision (the full set of information available was not revealed to them), whereas in the present studies they knew exactly what information was available. This structured presentation of information in the present study could have helped older adults organize their information processing. Second, Hershey, et al. (2003) had participants make multiple decisions with the same domain (investing in a retirement account) and in the current studies only a single decision was made. This shaped the way that each study operationalized information processing strategies; Hershey, et al. (2003) examined information processing scripts, whereas the present study focused on information search organization. Third, the current studies imposed a stressor on the participants where the Hershey study did not. It may be that had Hershey, et al. imposed processing restrictions or induced stress they would have found similar results. That said, both studies confirm that older adults have adapted to declines in basic abilities by relying on experience and knowledge to adapt to declines in basic cognitive abilities.

The findings from the present study raise questions about the effects that stress has on decision making. It is likely that the time constraints did induce a certain level of stress. In real life decisions that are time pressured, the stress that results from the situation can lead individuals to change their decision styles. Keinan (1987) found that stress did influence information processing and strategy use in a sample of young adults. Furthermore, compared to selecting an apartment, many of the decisions that older and even younger individuals face are often high stress or high conflict, such as selecting a treatment for cancer (Ferrell, et al., 2003) or deciding to place a loved one in a long-term care facility (McAuley and Travis, 2000). In these stressful situations, individuals may find themselves overwhelmed and conflicted over the decision at hand. Janis and Mann (1977) maintain that the severity of threat is linked to decision behavior such that the greater the threat the more likely it is that stress will impair decision processes. It may lead them to (a) make suboptimal decisions (b) allow others to make the decision for them rather than them working with others to make the decision or them making it for themselves or (c) avoid making a decison. Given this is it important to understand how stress impacts older adults' decision making processes and the outcomes of their decisions.

Limitations and Future Directions

The present study is limited in several ways. First, only one decision domain, selecting an apartment, was examined. It is possible that the findings would differ had another domain, such as medical treatment selection or an emotionally salient decision, had been used (Blanchard-Fields, Mienaltowski, and Seay 2007). Future studies should expand the number of decision domains included. Second, although it is likely that the time pressure did induce stress; it is not clear what would have happened in the time limits had been more stringent or if the decision task itself invoked stress. Would older adults continue to use the same strategies and heuristics for problem solving? Future studies should continue to examine the role of stress in information processing. Finally, the present study does not allow us to fully understand the role of basic cognitive abilities in decision making and how they can be compensated for or overcome. Future research should continue to focus on the role of basic abilities such as attention, executive function, and memory.

The importance of these findings for examinations of the everyday competence of older adults is fourfold. First, these findings are relevant to many decisions that are made under time pressures and/or time constraints on information processing. Time limits are inherent to the pace of everyday events, deadlines imposed by businesses, government, family, friends or colleagues, many of whom become impatient with the decision makers indecisiveness. However, these findings suggest that older adults adapted and did not lower their decision criteria leading to less optimal decisions. Second, the findings documented the strategy shifts that enabled older adults to adapt to the contexts of complex cognitive processes. The use of multiple markers for cognitive performance showed typical age-related declines for basic processes and highlighted effects for age and experimental conditions that indicate adaptive strategies. Third, these findings linked time to decision and information use to meta-memory measures. These links showed how objective task performance was related to how older adults felt about their cognitive abilities. Overall, the combined findings confirm that older adults are adaptive and can compensate for or overcome limitations in their basic information processing abilities when making complex real-world decisions. This information can be used to help develop aids that will assist older adults with complex decisions that have to be made under time pressure.

References

Allaire, J. C., and Marsiske, M. (2002). Well and ill defined measures of everyday cognition: Relationship to older adults' intellectual ability and functional status. *Psychology and Aging 17*(1), 101-115.

Anders, T. R., Fozard, J. L., and Lillyquist, T.D. (1972). Effects of age upon retrieval from short-term memory. *Developmental Psychology, 6*, 214-217.

Baltes, P. B., and Baltes, M. M. (1990). Psychological perspectives on successful aging: The model of selective optimization with compensation. In P. B. Baltes and M. M. Baltes (Eds.), *Successful aging: Perspectives from the behavioral sciences* (pp. 1–34). New York: Cambridge University Press.

Benson, L. III., and Beach, L. R. (1996). The effects of time constraints on the prechoice screening of decision options. *Organizational Behavior and Human Decision Processes, 67*, 222-228.

Blanchard-Fields, F., Mienaltowski, A., and Seay, R. (2007). Age differences in everyday problem solving effectiveness: Older adults select more effective strategies for interpersonal problems. *Journals of Gerontology: Series B: Psychological Sciences and Social Sciences, 62*, 61-64.

Böckenholt, U. and Hynan, L. S. (1994). Caveats on a process-tracing measure and a remedy. *Journal of Behavioral Decision Making, 7*, 103-117.

Burton, C., Strauss, E., Hultsch, D., and Hunter, M. (2006). Cognitive functioning and everyday problem solving in older adults. *Clinical Neuropsychologist, 20*(3), 432-452.

Cerella, J. (1990). Aging and information processing rate. In J.E. Birren and K.W. Schaie (Eds.) *Handbook of the Psychology of Aging*, (pp. 201-221). San Diego, CA: Academic Press.

Cacioppo, J. T., Petty, R.E., and Kao, C.F. (1984). The efficient assessment of need for cognition. *Journal of Personality Assessment, 48*, 306-307.

Charness, N., Kelley, C., Bosman, E., and Mottram, M. (2001). Word-processing training and retraining: Effects of adult age, experience, and interface. *Psychology and Aging, 16*(1), 110-127.

Crook, T. H. and Larrabee, G. J. (1992). Normative data on a self-rating scale for evaluating memory in everyday life. *Archives of Clinical Neuropsychology, 7*, 41-51

Daneman, M. and Carpenter, P. A. (1980). Individual differences in working memory and reading. *Journal of Verbal Learning and Verbal Behavior, 19*, 450-466.

Denney, N. W. (1985). A review of life span research with the twenty questions task: A study of problem solving ability. *International Journal of Aging and Human Development, 21*(3), 161-173.

Denney, N. W. (1989). Everyday problem solving: Methodological issues, research findings, and a model. In Poon, L. W., Rubin, D. C., and Wilson, B. A. (Eds.), *Everyday cognition in adulthood and late life* (pp.330-351). New York: Cambridge University Press.

Denney, N. W., and Pearce, K. A. (1989). A developmental study of practical problem solving in adults. *Psychology and Aging, 4*(4), 438-442.

Denney, N. W., Tozier, T. L., and Schlotthauer, C. A. (1992). The effect of instructions on age differences in practical problem solving. *Journals of Gerontology, 47*(3), 142-145.

Edland, A. (1994). Time pressure and the application of decision rules: Choices and judgements among multiattribute alternatives. *Scandanavian Journal of Psychology, 35*(3), 281-291.

Edland, A., and Svenson, O. (1993). Judgment and decision making under time pressure: Studies and findings. In Ola Svenson and A. John Maule (Eds.), *Time Pressure and Stress in Human Judgment and Decision Making*. New York: Plenum Press.

Ferrell, B. R., Chu, D. Z. J., Wagman, L., Juarez, G., Borneman, T., Cullinane, C.,et al. (2003). Patient and surgeon decision making regarding surgery for advanced cancer. *Oncology Nursing Forum, 30(6)*, E106-E114.

Friedman, D., Nessler, D., Johnson, R., Ritter, W., and Bersick, M. (2008). Age-related changes in executive function: An event-related potential (ERP) investigation of task-switching. *Aging, Neuropsychology, and Cognition, 15*(1), 1-34.

Gigerenzer, G., and Selten, R. (2001). *Bounded rationality: The adaptive toolbox*. Cambridge, MA: MIT Press.

Hartley, A. A. (1990). The cognitive ecology of problem-solving. In L.W. Poon, D.C. Rubin and B.A. Wilson (Eds.), *Everyday cognition in adulthood and later life* (pp.300-329). Cambridge, England: Cambridge Univ. Press.

Hartley, A. A., and Anderson, J. W. (1983). Task complexity and problem-solving performance in younger and older adults. *Journal of Gerontology, 38*(1), 72-77.

Hershey, D. A., Jacobs-Lawson, J. M. and Walsh, D. (2003). Influences of age and training on script development. *Aging, Neuropsychology, and Cognition, 10,* 1-19.

Hershey, D. A., Walsh, D. A., Read, S. J. and Chulef, A. S. (1990). The effects of expertise on financial problem solving: Evidence for goal directed problem solving scripts. *Organizational Behavior and Human Decision Processes, 46*, 77-101.

Janis, I. L. and Mann, L. (1977). *Decision Making: A Psychological Analysis of Conflict, Choice and Commitment.* New York: Free Press.

Johnson, M. (1990). Age differences in decision making: A process methodology for examining strategic information processing. *Journals of Gerontology, 45*(2), 75-78.

Johnson, M. M. S. (1993). Thinking about strategies during, before and after making a decision. *Psychology and Aging, 8*, 231-241.

Johnson, M. M. S. (1997). Individual differences in the voluntary use of a memory aid during decision making. *Experimental Aging Research, 23*, 33-43.

Johnson, M., and Drungle, S. (2000). Purchasing over-the-counter medications: The influence of age and familiarity. *Experimental Aging Research, 26*(3), 245-261.

Johnson, M. S. and Ryan, M. (2003). Influence of OTC labeling on older adult decision making. *Journal of Pharmaceutical Marketing and Management. 15*, 37-52.

Keinan, G. (1987). Decision making under stress: Scanning of alternatives under controllable and uncontrollable threats. *Journal of Personality and Social Psychology, 52*(3), 639-644.

Korchin, S. J. and Basowitz, H. (1957) Age difference in verbal learning. *Journal of Abnormal and Social Psychology, 54,* 64-69.

Lawton, M. P., Kleban, M. H., Dean, J., Rajagopal, D., and Parmelee, P. A. (1992). The Factorial generality of brief positive and negative affect measures. *Journal of Gerontology: Psychological Sciences, 47*, P228-P237.

Maule, A., Hockey, G. R., and Bdzola, L. (2000). Effects of time-pressure on decision making under uncertainty: Changes in affective states and information processing strategy. Acta *Psychologica, 104*(3), 283-301.

Maule, A. J., and Svenson, O. (1993). Theoretical and empirical approaches to behavioral decision making and their relation to time constraints. In O. Svenson and A. J. Maule (Eds.), *Time Pressure and Stress in Human Judgment and Decision Making,* New York: Plenum Press.

McAuley, W. J., and Travis, S. S. (2000). Factors influencing level of stress during the nursing home decision process. *Journal of Clinical Geropsychology, 6*(4), 269-278.

McDowd, J. M., and Shaw, R. J. (2000). Attention and aging: A functional perspective. In Clark, F. I. M., and Salthouse, T. A. (Eds.), *The Handbook of Aging and Cognition*, Malwah, NJ Lawrence Earlbaum Associates.

Murphy, M. D., and Puff, C. R. (1982). Free Recall: Basic methodology and analyses. In C. R.Puff (Ed.), *Handbook of research methods in human memory and cognition* (pp. 99-128). San Diego, CA: Academic Press.

Payne, J. W., Bettman, J. R., and Johnson, E. J. (1993). *The Adaptive Decision Maker.* Cambridge: Cambridge University Press.

Riggle, E. D. B., and Johnson, M. M. S. (1997). Age difference in political decision-making: Strategies for evaluating political candidates. *Political Behavior, 18*, 99-118.

Perlmutter, M. (1988). Cognitive potential throughout life. In J.E. Birren and V.L. Bengtson (Eds.), *Emergent Theories of Aging* (pp. 247-268). New York: Springer Publishing.

Salthouse, T. A. (1984). Effects of age and skill in typing. *Journal of Experimental Psychology: General, 113*, 345-371.

Salthouse, T. A. (1991). *Theoretical perspectives on cognitive aging.* Hillsdale NJ: Lawrence Erlbaum Assoc.

Salthouse, T. A. (1992). Working-memory mediation of adult age differences in integrative reasoning. *Memory and Cognition, 20*, 413-423.

Salthouse, T. (2000). Aging and measures of processing speed. *Biological Psychology*, *54*(1), 35-54.

Sheppard, L., and Vernon, P. (2008). Intelligence and speed of information-processing: A review of 50 years of research. *Personality and Individual Differences*, *44*(3), 535-551.

Shipley, W. C. (1967). *Shipley Institute of Living Scale.* Western Psychological Services.

Simon, H. A. (1955) On a class of skew distribution functions. Biometrika 42, 425-439.

Simon, H.A. (1967). The logic of heuristic decision making. In N. Rescher (Ed.), The logic of decision and action (pp. 1-20). Pittsburgh: The University of Pittsburgh.

Stine-Morrow, E., Parisi, J., Morrow, D., and Park, D. (2008). The effects of an engaged lifestyle on cognitive vitality: A field experiment. *Psychology and Aging*, *23*(4), 778-786.

Tranter, L., and Koutstaal, W. (2008). Age and flexible thinking: An experimental demonstration of the beneficial effects of increased cognitively stimulating activity on fluid intelligence in healthy older adults. *Aging, Neuropsychology, and Cognition*, *15*(2), 184-207.

Willis, S., Tennstedt, S., Marsiske, M., Ball, K., Elias, J., Koepke, K., et al. (2006). Long-term effects of cognitive training on everyday functional outcomes in older adults. *Journal of the American Medical Association*, *296*(23), 2805-2814.

In: New Directions in Aging Research
Editor: Ruby R. Brougham, pp. 145-166
ISBN 978-1-60741-976-1
© 2009 Nova Science Publishers, Inc.

Chapter 8

Future Time Perspective: Health, Income, and Age

Ruby R. Brougham*[*1] and Richard S. John[2]
[1]Chapman University, Orange, California, USA
[2]University of Southern California, Los Angeles, California, USA

Abstract

The current chapter reviews the relationship between future time perspective, income, health, and age. It is proposed that future time perspective, that is, how future experiences and consequences are evaluated and compared to the present, is one critical factor for understanding decision-making. Many personal decisions involve consequences (cost and benefits) that unfold over time. The current chapter focuses on health and financial decisions. Promoting preventive health behaviors and retirement savings is critical to the well-being of all Americans given the demographic trend in the United States toward a larger number of older adults using social services (e.g., Social Security and Medicare) and fewer working adults to pay for those services. Preventive health decisions (e.g., exercise, nutrition, and tobacco use) and financial decisions involve a trade-off between benefits (e.g., taking a vacation) and costs (e.g., depleting a savings account). Furthermore many of the trade-offs for preventive health and financial decisions involve an immediate benefit (e.g., eating dessert now) versus a delayed cost (gaining weight later) or an immediate cost (e.g., inconvenience and time to exercise) versus a delayed benefit (e.g., better cardiovascular health). The chapter reviews the fundamental concepts of intertemporal choice, time discounting, and related empirical research. New and emerging areas of research in future time perspective including future representation of events, age and life events, and emotion are discussed. In particular, the important role of age in future time perspective is identified and discussed. Future applications of research with an emphasis on specific determinants (e.g., anxiety) that tip decisions toward greater concern for future versus present consequences are reviewed.

[*] Correspondence concerning this article should be addressed to Ruby Brougham Chapman University, Department of Psychology, Orange, California 92866 Electronic mail may be sent to brougham@chapman.edu

Introduction

The population of the United States is aging. In 1940 only 6.9% of the population was over 65, today 12.6% are over 65, by 2030 about 20% of the population will be over 65, and the population over 85 will quadruple in size (U.S. Administration on Aging, 2008). This change in demographics is the result of two trends: declining fertility and a steady increase in life expectancy (National Center for Health Statistics, 2007). One significant consequence of these trends is a marked reduction in labor force participation. Although, one might expect that longer life expectancy would lead to longer working careers, this has not occurred. Instead the median age for retirement in the United States is 61 (Gendell, 2008). Therefore, it is expected in the next few decades that the number of employees paying taxes relative to the number of retirees who are drawing retirement benefits will decline and fewer financial resources will be available for social security and health services (The Organisation for Economic Co-operation and Development, 2001). Thus, the change in labor force participation, due to an aging population, has important implications for sustaining our current social services for older Americans.

In the next few decades, Americans will be confronted with a number of challenges pertaining to the well-being of older adults. First, aging populations are marked by a higher prevalence of chronic disease (e.g., cancer, cardiovascular, and diabetes). In 2004 the Centers for Disease Control and Prevention reported that chronic disease affects 90 million Americans and accounts for 70% of all deaths. Furthermore, for older adults, chronic diseases are often associated with disability, reduced quality of life, and increased health care costs (Centers for Disease Control and Prevention and the Merck Company Foundation, 2007).

The health care costs for older adults are substantial. Chronic disease accounts for about 95% of health care expenditures for older adults and in 2005, one-third of United States health care costs (336 billion) were spent on health care for older adults (Centers for Disease Control and Prevention and the Merck Company Foundation, 2007). Currently, people over the age of 65 spend 12% of their income on health care, while those under the age of 65 spend 2% of their income on health care (Desmond, Rice, Cubanski, and Neuman, 2007). Furthermore, future retirees will receive most of their health care coverage through Medicare rather than private insurance (Hoffman, Klees, and Curtis, 2008). Medicare insurance has become more difficult to fund. In 1950 there were 16 workers for each Medicare recipient; in contrast it is estimated that in 2015 there will be less than 3 workers for each Medicare recipient (Social Security Administration, 2000). Thus, with reduced labor force participation, our ability to continue to pay for the health care costs for an increasing number of older adults will be unsustainable.

A second major challenge for an aging population is retirement income. Retirement savings, pensions, and social security are the common sources of retirement income (Hartmann and Lee, 2003). Many retirees also continue to work in some form of employment, such as part-time work, for additional income (Shultz, 2003). However, many individuals do not have sufficient savings for retirement (Lusardi and Mitchell, 2007). For example, the Retirement Confidence Survey (Helman, Greenwald, VanDerhei and Copeland, 2007) found that 43% of workers age 55 and older had less than $43,000 in retirement savings (excluding the value of their primary residence). Furthermore, less than half of all workers participate in a retirement plan and 31% expect Social Security to be a major source of retirement income. Since Social Security benefits are expected to exceed Social Security resources by 2017 and be completely depleted by 2041, it remains uncertain as to whether Social Security will be a viable resource for future retirees (Social Security Administration, 2008). Thus, given current retirement savings rates and the potential for Social Security benefits to be depleted, many older adults will have insufficient funds for their retirement years.

Challenge also brings opportunity. Baby boomers (those born between 1946 and 1964) are the next generation to enter retirement. This generation of retirees expects more from retirement than past generations and they place a high value on maintaining health (American Association of Retired Persons, 2004). Past studies suggest that disability can be postponed or prevented by adopting healthier lifestyles (e.g., Chakravarty, Hubert, Lingala, and Fries, 2008; Hubert, Bloch, Oehlert and Fries, 2002; Wannamethee, Ebrahim, Papacosta, and Shaper, 2005). To a large extent chronic diseases are preventable. Poor health and disability are not an inevitable consequence of aging. People who are physically active, eat a healthy diet, do not use tobacco, and practice other healthy behaviors significantly reduce their risk for chronic diseases and disability (U.S. Department of Health and Human Services, 2002)

The increased life expectancy of the baby boom generation reflects, in part, our success in controlling infectious disease and acute illness, but public health promotion must now focus on quality of life issues and well-being in old age. In particular, the prevention of chronic disease (e.g. heart disease, diabetes) would substantially improve the quality of life in old age. Many individuals who are part of the baby boom generation are healthier, have greater education, have greater wealth, and can expect greater longevity than past cohorts (Manton, Gu and Lamb, 2006; Metlife Mature Market Institute, 2007). This generation also has greater diversity in race, wealth, and health than previous retirees (Eggebeen and Sturgeon, 2006; United States Bureau of the Census, 2007). If health can be maintained and we can successful compresses morbidity, that is, reduce the length of time that people spend disabled in old age, then we can reduce our medical expenditures and increase labor force participation at older ages. Currently, disability is one of the primary reasons for early retirement (Karpansalo, Kauhanen, and Lakka, 2005; Lund and Villadsen, 2005).

The baby boom generation is also the first generation to retire that will be primarily dependent on defined contribution (e.g. 401k) plan rather than a defined benefit plan[1] for retirement funds (Korczyk, 2008). In a defined contribution plan, the employee rather than the employer is responsible for managing the employee's retirement funds. This allows the employee maximum flexibility for investing retirement money and managing the risk involved with these investments. However, if employees underestimate their longevity or future consumption needs (such as health care), or overestimate their resources they may outlive their retirement money (Korczyk, 2008). Thus, retirement planning has become complex and requires long-term planning and education.

Although workers report anxiety regarding sufficient retirement funding, only 47% of all workers had completed a retirement needs calculation to find out 1) how much income they will need in retirement and 2) how much current income they will need to save to meet their retirement goals (Helman, Greenwald, VanDerhei and Copeland, 2007). Thus, worry about retirement does not translate into workers taking action to become better informed about their retirement needs. This anxiety seems well founded given that the median balance in 401k accounts for workers approaching retirement is only $60,000 and other savings beyond employee-sponsored plans is minimal (Munnell, Golub-Sass, Soto, and Webb, 2008). Furthermore, the National Retirement risk index (2006) reports that 40% of the baby boomers are “at risk” of being unable to maintain their current standard of living in retirement and 36% of workers 55 and older report they will only have sufficient funds to cover basic needs in retirement (Munnell, et al., 2008; Helman, et al., 2007). Clearly, Americans need to increase their rate of saving for retirement.

Although we know that retirement planning and saving are fundamental to having sufficient retirement funds, less is known about people’s motivation to save for retirement. Similarly, while a healthy lifestyle and preventive health behaviors including early detection practices (e.g., mammograms) are fundamental to avoiding chronic diseases, relatively little is known about why people decide to enact healthy behaviors in their daily lives. It is clear that a critical knowledge gap exists in understanding the motivations underlying health and retirement savings decisions. In order to develop and effectively target interventions for preventative health and retirement savings behaviors, a better understanding of motivation is necessary.

In an effort to promote preventive health behaviors and increase retirement savings many studies focus on education (e.g., Clark, d’Ambrosio, McDermed, and Sawant, 2003; Holland, Greenberg, Tidwell, and Newcomer, 2003). Clearly, education increases 1) people’s understanding of the importance of healthy lifestyles (e.g., exercising, eating nutritious foods) and retirement savings, and 2) people’s understanding of how to enact those procedures. Knowledge is an important tool for making decisions that lead to better health and sufficient retirement savings in old age. However, knowledge alone does not alter decision-making. We propose that a better understanding of future time perspective, that is, how future experiences and consequences are evaluated and compared to the present, will be one critical factor for understanding motivation. The ability to make accurate predictions about their future is based upon the ability to identify and evaluate the current and future consequences of actions. If we can understand the factors that influence predictions about the future, then we can guide individuals toward decisions that have a higher likelihood of greater well-being in old age.

The purpose of the current chapter is to explore the role of future-time perspective in decision-making. Future time perspective encompasses cognitive processes (e.g., planning, regulation of behavior), emotion (e.g., anxiety) and motivation (e.g., values and goals). Many conceptualizations of future time perspective have been used to explain and study how future consequences are evaluated and compared to immediate consequences. One of the first was the discounted utility model (Samuelson, 1937) that introduced the discount rate. The discount rate is a single numerical value that reflects an individual’s trade-off between what is forgone in the present versus what will be gained in the future. For example, one might be willing to forgo $500 of income per month now in exchange for $1,500 per month additional income after retirement. This model is widely used in the economic literature and has been used to measure discount rates for money, obesity, health behaviors, alcohol use, heroin use, and smoking (Bickel, Odum, and Madden 1999; Chabris, Laibson, Morris, Schuldt, and Taubinsky, 2008; Chapman, 2005: Chapman, 1996; Harrison, Lau, and Williams, 2002;

Huston and Finke, 2003; Komlos, Smith and Bogin 2004; Petry, Bickel, and Arnett, 1998; Petry, 2001)

Kurt Lewin (1951) proposed another early conceptualization of future time perspective. He defined future time perspective as the importance an individual attaches to the future that is informed by both current and past actions. Nuttin (1964) expanded on Lewin's ideas and proposed that motivation is largely determined by perception of the future. Currently, this theoretical framework is predominately operationalized by judgments about 1) the importance of the present compared to the future and 2) preference for thinking about the present or future. This framework is widely used in the psychological literature and has been used to measure a wide variety of behaviors including: risky health behaviors, exercise behaviors, retirement savings, and proenvironmental behaviors (Hall and Fong, 2003; Hershey and Mowen, 2000; Jacobs-Lawson and Hershey 2005; Keough, Zimbardo, and Boyd, 1999; Strathman, Gleicher, Boninger, and Edwards, 1994).

The current chapter begins with a brief review of intertemporal choice and time discounting. The remainder of the chapter explores the relationship between future time perspective and future representation of events, age and life events, and emotion. The chapter ends with a discussion of future directions for research that focuses on age differences in future time perspective.

Future Time Perspective

Intertemporal Choice

Intertemporal choice has been recognized as an important component of most consequential decisions (e.g., Lowenstein, Read and Baumeister, 2003). People often have to make intertemporal choices, that is, deciding among decision alternatives where the cost and benefits of each decision alternative is present at different times. Many decisions involve making a choice between a smaller more immediate benefit and a larger delayed benefit. For example, individuals choose between saving money for retirement or spending that money now. If they decide to spend their money now, then they will enjoy the short-term benefits of greater discretionary income (e.g., a ski trip to Tahoe) and they will suffer the consequences of insufficient retirement funds (e.g., insufficient funds to pay bills) later in their lives. Conversely, if individuals decide to save for retirement now they will have to live more frugally (e.g., inexpensive vacation, such as camping at the local mountains) but they will have the benefit of retirement funds (e.g., sufficient fund to pay bills) later in their lives. Thus, in order to make an informed intertemporal decision a person must: 1) understand the current cost and benefits of the decision, 2) understand the future cost and benefits of the decision, and 3) understand the trade-offs or compromises between the decision cost and benefits that will need to be made.

Discounted utility has been the primary theoretical model for quantifying intertemporal choice (Fredrick, Loewenstein and O'Donoghue, 2002). A basic assumption of the discounted utility model is that people choose a decision alternative based on their belief that a particular decision alternative relative to other decision alternatives will provide them with greater satisfaction or pleasure. Within the discounted utility framework, time discounting is the construct that captures preferences for more immediate benefits and more delayed costs. The following section of the chapter reviews time discounting.

Time Discounting

Conceptually, time discounting follows the traditional economic model of discounted utility that is commonly used in calculating the present value of alternatives involving costs and benefits that are distributed across time. As discussed by (Read and Read, 2004) the discount factor, δ, is represented as:

$$\delta = \left(\frac{x_1}{x_2}\right)^{(1/(t_1-t_2))}$$

where x_1 and x_2 are benefits that will be received at times t_1 and t_2. The discount factor can be estimated by finding a point of indifference, the point where the additional benefits received are large enough to compensate for the increased time delay. Thus, the discount factor allows for 1) a comparison of the cost and benefits of a decision over time, and 2) reflects the value the placed on the present versus the future. For example, if an individual equates the benefits of $100 received right now to the benefit of a $125 received a year from now, then this individual's discount factor is .80 and the annual discount rate would be 20%. Thus, this individual has expressed a positive discount rate, meaning that the delayed benefit must be increased by $25, to a total value of $125, to make the delayed value equivalent to the present benefit of $100.

One assumption of the discounted utility model is that discount rates are used to value delayed benefits over time (Fredrick, Loewenstein and O'Donoghue, 2002). For example, if $100 is worth 20% less if delayed one year, then the $100 should be worth an additional 20% less, a total of 40% less, if delayed for two years. One consistent finding for monetary outcomes is that people often report a positive discount rate placing greater value on current monetary outcomes than future monetary outcomes (e.g., Thaler, 1981). This result may be explained by people's response to uncertainty about the future and interest rates. For example, there is some chance that the promised $125 will not be received in a year; thus, it is less risky to accept $100 now. Discount rates may also be affected be the fact that $100 deposited into a bank savings account would earn interest and that a $100 loan would require payment of interest.

Discount Rates for Health and Money

The empirical results of discount rates for health and money are predominately high, at times 100% or more (Frederick, Loewenstein, and O'Donoghue, 2002). A high discount rate reflects the loss of a large percentage of value for a future outcome because of a time delay.

Thus, the research on time discounting concludes that most people place a large premium on the current benefits of health and money. However, some variability in discount rates has been found with several studies reporting zero and negative discount rates (Chapman and Coups, 1999; Ganiats, et al., 2000; Loewenstein, 1987; Van der Pol and Cairns, 2000). A zero discount rate indicates that a person rates the current and future benefits of health or money as having the same value, however, if a person has a negative discount rate then they place a premium on the future. For example, people who are present-oriented regarding health (have a high discount rate and thus place a high premium on the current benefits of their decisions) may smoke in order to reduce anxiety. In contrast, people who are future-oriented regarding health (have a lower discount rate and thus place a high premium on future benefits of their decisions) may consistently go to the gym in order to improve cardiovascular health and avoid a heart attack later in life. In the above health example, those with a high discount rate are more willing to engage in current health damaging behaviors with minimal concern for the future, while those with lower discount rates place greater value on future outcomes and are willing to endure short-term costs in exchange for larger benefits in the future.

Past research also suggests that discount rates are 1) higher for smaller benefits than larger benefits, and 2) higher for shorter time delays than longer time delays (Ainslie and Haslam, 1992; Chapman, 1996; Green, Myerson and McFadden, 1997; Read and Loewenstein, 2000). For example, Brougham and John (2007) found young adults (mean age = 20) who imagined themselves in poor health had the following discount rates for the future benefit of perfect health: 1) a 1 year delay for 1 year benefit of perfect health was discounted at 354%, 2) a 2 year delay for a 2 year benefit of perfect health was discounted at 70%, and 3) a 8 year delay for a 4 year benefit of perfect health was discounted at 39%. Thus, young adults preferred the shortest time delay and the smallest health benefit.

The preference for short time delays and smaller benefits may result from young adults' beliefs that the likelihood of obtaining a future benefit decreases over time. Therefore, a premium is placed on smaller immediate benefit because of a perceived higher chance of realization compared to delayed larger benefits that may never occur.

Past research also suggests that discount rates are higher for benefits than for costs (Hesketh, 2000; Lowenstein, 1987; Thaler, 1981). For example, a $100 benefit received right now is equal to $200 benefit received in one year (a 100% discount rate), and a loss of $100 right now is equal to a loss of $150 in one year (50% discount rate). In general, people are more sensitive to costs than benefits (Tversky and Kahneman, 1981).

A different pattern of time discounting preferences emerges for a singular vs. a sequence of decision outcomes. For decisions with a sequence of outcomes, research results indicate a preference for increasing sequences over decreasing sequences even when the overall benefits across the time periods was equivalent. A number of studies have found this effect for sequences of varying levels of income and pain, and varying desirability of dinners and vacations (Chapman, 2000; Loewenstein and Prelec, 1993; Loewenstein and Sicherman, 1991). For example, Chapman (2000) found that for hypothetical levels of headache pain, gradually decreasing levels of pain were preferred to gradually increasing levels of pain, even though the total headache pain experienced over the time sequence was identical. Thus, for time sequences people often express a negative discount rate, a preference for improving sequences over worsening sequences.

In sum, the results of past research in the domains of money and health using the time discounting framework suggests the following: 1) discount rates are predominately high, at times 100% or more, 2) discount rates are higher for smaller benefits than larger benefit, 3) discount rates are higher for shorter time delays than longer time delays, 4) discount rates are higher for benefits than for costs, and 5) discount rates are negative for improving sequences of money or health. Although past studies show a consistent pattern of time discounting preferences, less is known about the factors that influence future time perception. The next three sections of this chapter will review the role of future representation of events, age and life events, and emotions on future time perspective.

Representation of Future Events

Intertemporal decisions are often based on present needs and present needs are often perceived as more important than future needs (Loewenstein, 1996). One explanation for this preference is based on people's ability to imagine how decision consequences will affect their future welfare (Becker and Mulligan, 1997). Trope and Liberman's (2003) construal level theory suggests that the ability to imagine the future may be based upon mental representations of future events that change as a result of temporal proximity. Specifically, current needs that are salient are represented in concrete details while future needs are more likely to be represented by a few general abstract features (Trope and Liberman, 2003). For example, thoughts about a ski trip later this year may include concrete images and details, such as the exhilaration of skiing down the mountain, and the beauty of the snow capped mountains.

In contrast, thoughts about retirement thirty years into the future may be represented by an abstract goal, such as "having sufficient funds." Trope and Liberman (2003) also suggest that less information is available about the future, resulting in greater overconfident and less accurate predictions about the future. Thus, if the future consequences of a decision are made: 1) salient and concrete, and 2) the delayed benefit or cost is made sufficiently high, than a person may be willing to forgo present benefits for future benefits (Mischel, Ayduk, and Mendoza-Denton, 2003). Thus, saving for retirement would be more attractive option if individuals could vividly and concretely image their futures, such as touring Paris or being destitute and homeless.

Since age and life events provide individuals with greater experience and information, it is likely that age and life events influence future time perspective. In particular, the likelihood of decision outcomes and the value for those decision outcomes is likely to change as a result of age and life events. The next section of the chapter will review the relationship between age, life events, and future time perspective.

Age and Life Events

Some researchers have found age differences in future time perspectives (Read and Read, 2004; Green, Fry and Myerson, 1994). For example, Read and Read (2004) found that older adults reported higher discount rates than middle age and young adults. Specifically, older adults were found to prefer a shorter holiday now to a longer holiday later. Since, the older adult's perceived likelihood of death or illness is greater than the middle age or young adults, older adults would rather take a holiday now then wait until next year. Thus, older adult's perception of the future as uncertain due to illness or mortality is one possible explanation for the age differences in time discounting rates.

However, other research suggests a different developmental trajectory for time discounting. For example, Green, Fry and Myerson (1994) and Brougham and John (2007) found that young adults had greater discount rates than older adults. Thus, young adults expressed a stronger preference compared to older adults for immediate benefits versus delayed benefits. One potential explanation for this result is that younger adults are more impulsive than older adults. The slow maturation of the prefrontal cortex (Steinberg, 2008) and the lack of experience with life events may account for the greater impulsivity of younger adults. Impulsive individuals show a disregard for future consequences and are more likely to be involved in risk-taking behaviors (Granö, Virtanen, Vahtera, Elovainio, and Kivimäki, 2004). Within the time discounting framework, impulsivity is related to stronger preferences for options leading to smaller immediate benefits over options to wait for larger delayed benefits (Ainslie, 1975). The results of past research provide mixed support for the relationship between impulsivity and people's preference for immediate benefits (de Wit, Flory, Acheson, McCloskey, and Manuck, 2007; Reynolds, Ortengren, Richards, and de Wit, 2006; Richards, Zhang, Mitchell, and de Wit,1999). Furthermore, the relationship between impulsivity and adult age differences (young adults, middle-age. and older adults) in preference for immediate versus delayed benefits has not been systematically studied. Clearly, research is needed that examines the relationship between age differences, impulsivity, and time discounting.

Socioemotional selectivity theory (Carstensen, 1995) provides another perspective on age differences and future time perspective. The central tenet of socioemotional selectivity theory is that time perspective is bound by how much time an individual has left to live. Thus, older adults have a shorter future time perspective, while younger adults have a longer future time perspective. Furthermore, within the framework of socioemotional selectivity theory personal goals are prioritized in relation to time perspective. Thus, young adults pursue future oriented goals such as acquiring information and personal development, while older adults pursue present-oriented goals, such as having emotional meaningfully encounters and regulating emotions (e.g., avoiding negative states, intensifying positive states). Löckenhoff and Carstensen (2004) propose that specific age differences in information processing are the result of differences in future time perspective. Specifically, research suggests that older adults seek to regulate emotion by paying attention to and remembering positive information and avoiding negative information (Charles, Mather and Carstensen, 2003; Mather and Carstensen, 2005). This difference in information processing may result in poorer quality decisions for older adults. For example, in making health-related decisions older adults seek less information (e.g., Zwahr, Park and Shifren, 1999) are less likely to incorporate new information (e.g., Okun and Rice, 2001), and more likely to avoid making decisions than younger adults (e.g., Meyer, Russo and Talbot, 1995). Thus, a shorter future time perspective is associated with a reduction in the quality of information processing for decisions.

Experience with life events may be another explanation for the age differences found in future time perspective. Middle age and older adults are more likely to have had significant life experiences, such as marriage, being diagnosed with a chronic illness, becoming a parent, experiencing death of a family member, and being terminated from a job. Thus, middle age and older adults have more information about the consequences of decisions and should be better at estimating probabilities of future consequences resulting from a particular decision. The next section of the chapter examines the relationship between life events and future time perspective.

Liu and Aaker (2007) found that young adults differed in their time related preferences based on whether or not they had experienced the death of a significant person in their life. Specifically, young adults who had experienced the death of a significant person in their life were more likely to choose decision outcomes that incurred small short-term costs in exchange for a larger delayed benefit than young adults who had not experienced a death of a significant person in their life. For example, young adults who had experienced a death event allocated a greater percentage of a $400 tax refund to a long-term savings account rather than spend it. Furthermore, a preference for larger delayed benefits over smaller immediate benefits could be temporarily induced by asking young individuals to image the death of their best friend. Liu and Aaker (2007) propose that the experience of a death event may shift focus from the present to the future. While, the Liu and Aaker study provides support for the relationship between significant life experiences and time perception for young adults, there have been no studies reporting the impact of life experiences on the time perception of middle-age and older adults.Furthermore, it is unclear as to whether the experience of death event is unique or if other life experiences such as job and career changes, marriage and divorce, and having children would also shift time perspective from the present to the future.

Another explanation for age differences in future time perspective may be attributed to age related changes in reference points. Prospect theory suggests that outcomes resulting from a decision are evaluated as deviations from a reference point that normally represents the status quo (Kahneman, and Tversky, 1979). Kahneman and Tversky (1979) introduced prospect theory as a descriptive explanation of how people value gains and losses associated with a decision. For example, applied to health decisions, prospect theory suggests that potential changes in health are valued as either gains or losses relative to current health status (a fixed reference point). Empirical research is consistent with predictions from prospect theory utilizing a risk averse utility function for gains from the status quo (reference point) and a risk seeking utility function for losses from a reference point (Budescu and Weiss , 1987; Loewenstein, 1988; Tversky and Kahneman, 1992). Thus, the location of the reference point for health decisions partially determines whether health decision makers will be risk averse or risk seeking for particular positive outcomes. Since the reference point is normally associated with the status quo, it follows that age may play a particularly critical role in determining the location of the reference point.

It is expected that the location of the reference point will shift toward risk aversion as people age. Thus, potential future consequences would be viewed as gains from the reference point. For example, Happich and Mazurek (2002) found support for a correlation between health related quality of life and risk attitude. Specifically, experience with negative health conditions was related to increasing risk aversion in health decision making. Since the likelihood of negative health experiences increases with age, risk aversion is expected to increase with age.

Schwartz, Goldberg, and Hazen (2008) propose manipulating people's reference points to increase compliance to preventive health procedures by directing people to imagine their future health as they age. This manipulation results in a contrast effect where the smaller costs of a typical diagnostic procedure (e.g., inconvenience, time, money) are compared to the larger costs of a missed early diagnosis of cancer (reduced quality of life, reduced longevity, pain). Furthermore, Schwartz, Goldberg, and Hazen (2008) argue within the framework of prospect theory, that discount rates for deciding to endure diagnostic health procedures should be lower when individuals are induced to use a reference point of anticipated future health (e.g., poor health in old age) compared to a reference point reflecting current health. Schwartz, Goldberg, and Hazen (2008) report that the loss incurred due to a diagnostic procedure is smaller when using the reference point of poor health in old age than when using the reference point of current health status. Furthermore, using the reference point of poor health at old age, the gain incurred from early detection of cancer is much greater than the gain incurred using current health state. Shifts in reference points have not been systematically investigated. Greater research is needed to 1) identify age differences in reference points, and 2) assess the effects of reference point manipulations on future time perspective.

Emotions may also account for differences in time perspective. In response to an emotion, such as pleasure, short-term benefits (e.g., unprotected sexual encounter) may be more salient than long-term costs (e.g., sexually transmitted disease). In contrast, other emotions such as anxiety may shift focus to the future and make short-term costs (e.g., give up a vacation) relatively less important than long-terms benefits (e.g., adequate savings for retirement). The next section of the chapter will discuss the relationship between emotion and future time perspective.

Emotion

Emotion also plays a role in time perspective. Understanding current feelings and predicting how those feelings will change over time is an important aspect of decision-making. Rick and Lowenstein (2008) propose that both anticipated and immediate emotions play a role in defining future time perspective. Anticipated emotions are the emotions that one expects to experience as a result of a decision outcome. Anticipated emotions are personal forecasts of how one will feel in the future. For example, in deciding whether to take a vacation, one might imagine the pleasure of skiing down a mountain or the guilt and anxiety related to depleting a saving account for a ski trip.

Past research suggests that people have difficulty in accurately forecasting their future emotions (Chapman and Coups, 2006; Wilson and Gilbert, 2003). Kassam, Gilbert, Boston, and Wilson (2008) suggest that differences in time discounting may in part be attributed to an error in emotional forecasting know as future anhedonia. It is proposed that individuals erroneously use the status quo, how they currently feel about a decision outcome, to predict how they will feel in the future about a decision outcome. Since future outcomes are represented as general and abstract they produce less affect than current outcomes that are represented as concrete with specific details (Trope and Liberman, 2003). Thus, future decision outcomes are devalued because individuals underestimate the intensity of the pleasure or pain they will feel as a result of a cost or benefit in the future.

Lowenstein (1987) also proposed that savoring and dread augment emotional experience. For example, dread is experienced when one expects a negative consequence, such as physical pain. Since past research suggests that future consequences are devalued (Ainslie and Haslam, 1992), it would be expected that the delay of negative consequences (e.g., pain) would be preferred to the immediate realization of negative consequences (e.g., pain). However, Loewenstein (1987) found that individuals' preferred immediate physical pain to delayed physical pain. One explanation is that the emotional distress related to waiting and anticipating physical pain in the future is worse than experiencing pain immediately. In contrast, for a positive experience such as dinner at a fancy restaurant, individuals prefer to savor the anticipated positive consequence. Loewenstein (1987) found that anticipation of positive consequences (e.g., dinner at a fancy restaurant) results in a preference for delayed positive experiences rather than immediate positive experiences. Thus, positive and negative anticipated emotions may influence future time perspective.

Immediate emotions also play a role in time perspective. Immediate emotions are those experienced at the time of choice. For example, in deciding whether to undergo a preventive screening test, the decision maker may immediately experience feelings of fear and anxiety. Thus, immediately experienced feelings may change the value of the decision outcome and the change in value may result in a change in time preference.

Immediately experienced feelings may arise from visceral influences, such as hunger, sexual desire, and pain (Loewenstein, 1996). Furthermore, visceral influences may place an individual into a "hot" state that demands attention and directs individuals toward goal-oriented behaviors. While in a "hot" state, information in processed quickly and emotional processing dominates cognitive processing (Metcalfe and Mischel, 1999). Visceral factors often increase the value of an immediate benefit. Thus, individuals in "hot" states are prone to act impulsively and often overestimate the amount of time they will be in a "hot" state (Loewenstein, 2000). Chapman (2005) also found that time preference was strongly related to engaging in "hot" behaviors (e.g., smoking) but only weakly related to "cool" behaviors (e.g., flu vaccination).

Individuals also experience "hot-cold" empathy gaps (Loewenstein, 2005). Those who are in a "cool" state engage in deliberate cognitive processing (Metcalfe and Mischel, 1999) and underestimate the influence of "hot" state on their behavior when they are in a cool state (Loewenstein, 2005). This underestimation may be due in part to difficulty in remembering the "hot" state. For example, Read and Loewenstein (1999) found that individuals had difficulty remembering the experience of pain (placing their hand in cold water one week earlier) and required less compensation to repeat the pain experience than individuals who just completed the painful task.

Other immediate emotions may occur as an inseparable part of the decision, such as the "pain of paying" or the "joy of spending." For example, people who immediately experience the "pain of paying" for an item because the cost of the item is higher than expected or because they find spending money to be painful (e.g., they are tightwads) are deterred from immediate spending (Rick, Cryder, and Loewenstein,, 2008; Knutson, Rick, Wimmer, Prelec and Lowenstein, 2007). Thus, particular contextual factors and personality characteristics influence whether the immediate pain of paying will be greater than the perceived pleasure of spending.

Negative emotions such as worry and regret also influence future time perspective. Regret occurs as a consequence of a negative decision outcome (Zeelenberg, van Dijk, Manstead, and van der Plight, 1998). Furthermore, regret occurs when the responsibility for the negative decision outcome is clearly the decision maker's (Zeelenberg, van Dijk, Manstead, and van der Plight, 1998; Zeelenberg, van Dijk, Manstead, and van der Plight, 2000). The results of past studies found that focusing on feelings that would occur as a result of engage in a regrettable behavior (e.g., unsafe sexual practices) reduced people's engagement in that behavior (Richard, van der Plight, and de Vries, 1996). Thus, anticipated regret is dependent upon an understanding of post-decisional feelings (Zeelenberg, 1999). Furthermore, Chapman and Coups (2006) also found that feelings of regret were associated with changes in health behavior. Specifically, Chapman and Coups (2006) found that individuals who experienced greater regret over their decision to forgo a flu vaccination were more likely to accept a flu vaccination in the subsequent year than individuals who experienced less regret. In contrast, optimism for a health related outcome was associated with a shorter future time perspective (Berndsen, and Van der plight, 2001).

Anticipated anxiety results in worry. Differences in level of worry have been associated with behaviors that reflect differences in future time perspective (Cameron and Diefenbach, 2001; Chapman and Coups, 2006). For example, past research suggests that moderate levels of worry or anticipated anxiety are related to a greater likelihood of engaging in preventive health behaviors, such as cancer screening and flu vaccination (Chapman and Coups, 2006; Consedine, Magai, and Neugut, 2004; Consedine, Adjei, Ramirez, and McKiernan, 2008; Moser, McCaul, Peters, Nelson, and Marcus, 2007). Thus, people who are moderately worried about their health are more likely to exchange short-term costs (e.g., inconvenience, pain, time) of taking a preventive action for long-term benefits (e.g., early detection of cancer). However, high levels of anxiety that impair functioning are related to reductions in adherence to preventive health behaviors (Andersen, Smith, Meischke, Bowen, and Urban, 2003; Lerman and Schwartz, 1993, Miller, Fang, Manne, Engstrom and Daly, 1999). Furthermore, worry has been found to mediate the relationship between risk assessments (severity and likelihood) and preventive health behaviors (Cameron and Diefenbach, 2001; Chapman and Coups, 2006).

Clearly anticipated, immediate, and experienced emotion influence future time perspective. However, people have difficulty in extracting accurate information from their emotions. Specifically, they are inaccurate in forecasting future emotion, they have difficulty in understanding and regulating "hot" emotional states, and they suffer from "hot-cold" empathy gaps. Negative emotions such as worry and regret have been associated with behaviors that reflect greater future time perspective. Thus, behavioral interventions designed to change future time perspective are more likely to be successful in changing behavior when emotion is included as part of the intervention. For example, behavioral options (e.g. flu vaccination) are more attractive when emotions such as worry or regret are induced, resulting in greater focus on long-term advantages (e.g., prevention of sickness from the flu) and less concern about the short-term costs (e.g., cost, time, inconvenience).

Future Directions for Research

Current research has begun to investigate the important influence of individual difference variables (e.g., age, emotion) on time perspective. However, important questions about individual difference variables remain unanswered. In particular, identifying the nature of systematic age differences in future time perspective is one important gap in the time perspective literature. The few studies that have examined age differences in future time perspective report inconsistent results. Some studies report shorter time perspective for older adults than young and middle-age adults (e.g., Read and Read, 2004), while other studies report shorter time perspective for younger adults than older adults (Brougham and John 2007; Green, Fry, and Myerson, 1994). Potential explanations for the influence of age differences on future time perspective include impulsivity, time left in life, experience with life events, ability to enjoy consumption, and personal fertility (Ainslie, 1975; Carstensen, 1995; Trostel and Taylor, 2001; Rogers, 1994; Liu and Aaker, 2007). Thus, the proposed explanations for determinants of age differences in adult time discounting are varied and in need of further empirical research. Furthermore, a discovery of a general trajectory in future time perspective over the adult lifespan would be a potentially important and useful development.

The relationship between future time perspective and cognitive and emotional processing is another important emerging area of research. For example, Carstensen's socioemotional selectivity theory (1995) suggests that a shortened future time perspective motivates people to place greater priority on emotionally meaningful goals and on regulation of emotions. However, efforts to regulate emotion (e.g., ignoring negative information, paying attention to, and remembering positive information) may result in reductions in cognitive processing (e.g., seeking less information, difficulty integrating new information) that result in lower quality decisions.

Life events (e.g., marriage, death of a significant other) and people's ability to vividly represent future events may also influence time perspective. The longer life experience of older and middle age adults may translate into more realistic and concrete representations of future events than young adults' representations of the future. Thus, age differences in the representation of future events would be another avenue of future research.

Anticipated and experienced emotions of worry and regret are related to behaviors that reflect a longer future time perspective, such as engaging in health preventive measures (e.g., flu shot). However, few studies review the relationship between positive emotions (such as optimism and happiness) and future time perspective (Berndsen and van der Plight, 2001;

Drake and Duncan, 2008). Since older adults show a positivity effect, they pay attention to and remember positive information and often ignore negative information (Mather and Carstensen, 2003), it is important to understand the relationship between positive emotions and future time perspective. Thus, the relationship between positive emotions, future time perspective and age is another domain in need of further research.

Applications

In making decisions most individuals prefer to experience benefits in the present and costs in the future. For health promotion and savings behaviors, most costs are in the present and most benefits are in the future. For example, the costs of exercise behavior (time, inconvenience, and discomfort) are experienced in the present while the benefits (weight reduction, improvements in cardiovascular health) are experienced in the future. Thus, any single exercise session requires immediate costs but does not result in any immediately noticeable benefits.

Interventions that focus on changing behavior by presenting information on the long-term consequences of behavior (e.g., benefits) are unlikely to result in change because the cost are immediate and certain, while the benefits are delayed and uncertain. One alternative for behavioral interventions is to use knowledge-based interventions that focus on short-term cost and benefits.

For example, the immediate positive changes in physical health (e.g., mood enhancement) due to exercise should be identified and the short-term costs (e.g., loss of one-hour of time) of exercise should be realistically appraised.

Asymmetric paternalism (Loewenstein, Brennan and Volpp, 2007) is suggested as an alternative to traditional knowledge based interventions. Asymmetric paternalism is proposed as a set of policy reforms to guide those who are prone to making irrational decisions without harming those who make rational decisions. For example, to change behaviors for those individuals who are present oriented it would be necessary to change short-term incentives to guide individuals to better choices.

For example, most employees would accept having a free one-year gym membership (provided by company's health plan) with the provision that if the gym were not accessed at least 10 days per month the employee would have to pay a penalty. Since the gym membership is pre-paid, the employee's healthy behavior incurs no immediate financial cost, however, not going to the gym results in a future financial penalty. Thus, the proposed gym membership capitalizes on the individual's present bias.

Conclusion

Changing work force demographics, greater life expectancy, and an economic recession have increased the urgency of finding ways to intervene in lifestyles decision that lead to health and income problems in old age. Clearly, time perspective is an important variable in decision-making. In general, a longer future time perspective is associated with better quality decisions. A better understanding of the individual difference variables (e.g., age, emotion) that influence the trade-offs between immediate and future consequences has the potential to provide insight into how to target behavioral interventions to increase health promotion and savings behaviors.

References

Ainslie, G. (1975). Specious reward: A behavioral theory of impulsiveness and impulse control. *Psychological Bulletin, 82*(4), 463-496.

Ainslie, G. and Haslam, N. (1992). Hyperbolic discounting. In G. Loewenstein and J. Elster (Eds.), *Choice over time* (pp. 57-92). New York: Russell Sage Foundation.

American Association of Retired Persons. (2004). *The savings race.* AARP Bulletin Today.

Andersen, M. R., Smith, R. H., Meischke, H., Bowen, D., and Urban, N. (2003). Breast cancer worry and mammography use by women with and without a family history in a population-based sample. *Cancer Epidemiology, Biomakers and Prevention, 12*, 314-320.

Becker, G. S., and Mulligan, C. B. (1997). The endogenous determination of time preference. *Quarterly Journal of Economics, 112*(3), 729-758.

Berndsen, M., and van der Pligt, J. (2001). Time is on my side: Optimism in intertemporal choice. *Acta Psychologica,* 108, 173-186.

Bickel, W., Odum, A., and Madden, G. (1999). Impulsivity and cigarette smoking: delay discounting in current, never and ex-smokers. *Psychopharmacology, 146*(4), 447-454.

Brougham, R. R., and John, R. S. (2007). Age differences in preventive health decision. In P. W. O'Neal (Ed.), *Motivation of health behavior* (pp. 49-63). Hauppauge, NY: Nova Science Publishers, Inc.

Budescu, D. V., and Weiss, W. (1987). Reflection of transitive and intransitive preferences, a test of prospect theory. *Organizational Behavior and Human Decision Processes, 39*, 184–202.

Cameron, L. D., and Diefenbach, M. A. (2001). Responses to information about psychosocial consequences of genetic testing for breast cancer susceptibility: Influences of cancer, worry, and risk perceptions. *Journal of Health Psychology, 6*(1), 47-59.

Carstensen, L. L. (1995). Evidence for a life-span theory of socioeconomic selectivity. *Current Directions in Psychological Science, 4*(5), 151-162.

Centers for Disease Control and Prevention. (2004). *Chronic disease prevention.* Atlanta, GA: US Department of Health and Human Services, CDC, National Center for Chronic Disease Prevention and Health Promotion.

Centers for Disease Control and Prevention and the Merck Company Foundation. (2007). *The state of aging and health in America 2007.* Whitehouse Station, NJ: The Merck Company Foundation.

Chabris, C. F., Laibson, D., Morris, C. L., Schuldt, J. P., and Taubinsky, D. (2008). *Individual laboratory-measured discount rates predict field behavior* (NBER Working Paper No. 14720). Cambridge, MA: National Bureau for Economic Research.

Chakravarty, E. F., Hubert, H. B., Lingala, V. B., and Fries, J. F. (2008). Reduced disability and mortality among aging runners: A 21-year longitudinal study. *Archives of Internal Medicine, 168*(15), 1638-1646.

Chapman, G. B. (1996). Temporal Discounting and Utility for Health and Money. *Journal of Experimental Psychology: Learning, Memory and Cognition 22*(3), 771-791.

Chapman, G.B. (2000). Preferences for improving and declining sequences of health outcomes. *Journal of Behavioural Decision Making, 13*(2), 203-218.

Chapman, G. B. (2005). Short-Term Cost for Long-Term Benefit: Time Preference and Cancer Control. *Health Psychology 24*(4), 41-48.

Chapman, G. B., and Coups, E. J. (1999). Time preference and preventive health behavior. *Medical Decision Making, 19*(3), 307-314.

Chapman, G. B., and Coups, E. J. (2006). Emotions and preventive health behavior: Worry, regret, and influenza vaccination. *Health Psychology, 25*(1), 82-90.

Charles, S. T., Mather, M., and Carstensen, L. L. (2003). Aging and emotional memory: The forgettable nature of negative images for older adults. *Journal of Experimental Psychology: General, 132*, 310-324.

Clark, R. L., Ambrosio, M. B., McDermed, A. A., and Sawant, K. (2003). *Financial education and retirement savings*. Paper presented at the conference of the Federal Reserve System, Washington, DC.

Consedine, N. S., Magai, C., and Neugut, A. I. (2004). The contribution of emotional characteristics to breast cancer screening among women from six ethnic groups. *Preventive Medicine, 38*(1), 64-77.

Consedine, N. S., Adjei, B. A., Ramirez, P. M., and McKiernan, J. M. (2008). An object lesson: Source determines the relations that trait anxiety, prostate cancer worry, and screening fear hold with prostate screening frequency. *Cancer Epidemiology, Biomakers, and Prevention, 17*(7), 1631-1639.

Desmond, K. A., Rice, T., Cubanski, J., and Neuman, P. (2007). *The burden of out-of-pocket health spending among older versus younger adults: Analysis from the consumer expenditure survey, 1998-2003.* (Medicare Issue Brief Publication No. 7686). Menlo, CA: Kaiser Family Foundation.

de Wit, H., Flory, J. D., Acheson, A., McCloskey, M., and Manuck, S. B. (2007). IQ and nonplanning impulsivity are independently associated with delay discounting in middle-aged adults. *Personality and Individual Differences, 42*,111–121.

Drake, L., and Duncan, E. (2008). Time perspective and correlates of wellbeing. *Time and Society, 17*(1), 47-61.

Eggebeen, D. J., and Sturgeon, S. (2006). Demography of the baby boomers. In S. K. Whitebourne and S. L. Willis (Eds.), *The baby boomers grow up: Contemporary perspectives on midlife* (pp. 3-22). Mahwah, NJ: Lawrence Erlbaum Associates.

Evans, J. A. (2003). Awareness of long-term consequences as a factor in risky and prosocial behavior. *Dissertation Abstracts International: Section B: The Sciences and Engineering, 64*(4-B), 1888.

Frederick, S., Loewenstein, G. and O'Donoghue, T. (2002). Time discounting and time preference: A critical review. *Journal of Economic Literature. 40*(2), 351-401.

Ganiats, T. G., Carson, R. T., Hamm, R. M., Cantor, S.B., Sumner, W., Spann, S .J., et al. (2000). Population-based time preferences for future health outcomes. *Medical Decision Making 20*(3), 263-270.

Gendell, M. (2008). Older workers: increasing their labor force participation and hours of work. *Monthly Labor Review, 131*(1) 41-54.

Granö, N., Virtanen, M., Vahtera, J., Elovainio, M., and Kivimäki, M. (2004). Impulsivity as a predictor of smoking and alcohol consumption. *Personality and Individual Differences, 37*(8), 1693-1700.

Green, L., Fry, A. F., and Myerson, J. (1994). Discounting of delayed rewards: A life-span comparison. *Psychological Science, 5*(1), 33-36.

Green, L., Myerson, J., and McFadden, E. (1997). Rate of temporal discounting decreases with amount of reward. *Memory and Cognition, 25*(5),715-723.

Hall, P. A., and Fong, G. T. (2003). The effects of a brief time perspective intervention for increasing physical activity among young adults. *Psychology and Health, 18*(6), 685-706.

Happich, M., and Mazurek, B. (2002). Priorities and prospect theory. *The European Journal of Health Economics, 3*(1), 40-46.

Harrison, G. W., Lau, M. I., and Williams, M. B. (2002). Estimating individual discount rates in Denmark: A field experiment. *The American Economic Review, 92*(5), 1606-1617.

Hartmann, H., and Lee, S. (2003). *Social security: The largest source of income for both women and men in retirement* (IWPR Publication No: D455). Washington, DC: Institute for Women's Policy Research.

Helman, R., Greenwald, M., VanDerhei, J. and Copeland, C. (2007). *The retirement systems in transition: The 2007 retirement confidence survey* (EBRI Issue Brief No. 304). Washington, DC: Employee Benefit Research Institute.

Hesketh, B. (2000). Time perspective in career-related choices: Application of time-discounting principles. *Journal of Vocational Behavior, 57*(1), 62-84.

Hershey, D. A., and Mowen, J. C. (2000). Psychological determinants of financial preparedness for retirement. *The Gerontologist, 40*, 687-697.

Hoffman, E. D., Jr., Klees, B. S., and Curtis, C. A. (2008). *Brief Summaries of Medicare and Medicaid: Title XVIII and Title XIX of the Social Security Act as of November 1 2008.* Washington, DC: U. S. Department of Health and Human Services, Office of the Actuary, Centers for Medicare and Medicaid Services.

Holland, S. K., Greenberg, J., Tidwell, L., and Newcomer, R. (2003). Preventing disability through community-based health coaching. *Journal of American Geriatric Society, 51*, 265-269.

Hubert, H. B., Block, D. A., Oehlert, J. W., and Fries, J. F. (2002). Lifestyle habits and compression morbidity. *The Journals of Gerontology SeriesA: Biological Sciences and Medical Sciences, 57A*(6), M347-M351.

Huston, S. J., and Finke, M. S. (2003). Diet choice and the role of time preference. *Journal of Consumer Affairs, 37*(1), 143-160.

Jacobs-Lawson, J. M., and Hershey, D. A. (2005). Influence of future time perspective, financial knowledge, and financial risk tolerance on retirement saving behavior. *Financial Services Review, 14*, 331-344.

Kahneman, D., and Tversky, A. (1979). Prospect theory: An analysis of decision under risk. *Econometrica, 47*, 263-291.

Karpansalo, M., Kauhanen, J., and Lakka, T. (2005). Depression and early retirement: Prospective population based study in middle-aged men. *Journal of Epidemiology and Community Health, 59*(1) 70-74.

Kassam, K. S., Gilbert, D. T., Boston, A., and Wilson, T. D. (2008). Future anhedonia and time discounting. *Journal of Experimental Social Psychology, 44*(6), 1533-1537.

Keough, K. A., Zimbardo, P. G., and Boyd, J. N. (1999). Who's smoking, drinking, and using drugs? Time perspective as a predictor of substance use. *Basic and Applied Social Psychology, 21*, 149-164.

Komlos, J., Smith, P. K., and Bogin, B. (2004). Obesity and the rate of time preference: Is there a connection? *Journal of Biosocial Science, 32*(2), 209-219.

Korczyk, S. (2008). Who is ready for retirement, how ready, and how can we know? *AARP Public Policy Institute Research Report*. Washington, DC: AARP Public Policy Institute.

Knutson, B., Rick, S., Wimmer, G. E., Prelec, D,. and Loewenstein, G. (2007). Neural predictors of purchases. *Neuron, 53*(1), 147–156.

Lerman, C., and Schwartz, M. (1993). Adherence and psychological adjustment among women at high risk for breast cancer. *Breast Cancer Research and Treatment, 28*(2), 145-155.

Lewin, K. (1951) *Field theory in social science; selected theoretical papers.* D. Cartwright (Ed.). New York: Harper and Row.

Liu, W., and Aaker, J. (2007). Do you look to the future or focus on today? The impact of life experience on intertemporal decisions. *Organizational Behavior and Human Decision Processes. 102*(2), 212-225.

Löckenhoff, C. E., and Carstensen, L. L. (2004). Socioemotional selectivity theory, aging, and health: The increasingly delicate balance between regulating emotions and making tough choices. *Journal of Personality, 72*(6), 1395-1424.

Loewenstein, G. (1987). Anticipation and valuation of Delayed consequences. *Economy Journal, 97*, 666-684.

Loewenstein, G. (1988). Frames of mind in intertemporal choice. *Management Science, 34*, 200-214.

Loewenstein, G. (1996). Out of control: Visceral influences on behavior. *Organizational Behavior and Human Decision Processes, 65*, 272-292.

Loewenstein, G. (2000). Emotions in economic theory and economic behavior. *American Economic Review: Paper and Proceedings, 90*, 426-432.

Loewenstein, G. (2005). Hot-cold empathy gaps and medical decision making. *Health Psychology, 24*(4S), S49-S56.

Loewenstein, G., Brennan, T., and Volpp, K. G. (2007). Protecting people from themselves: Using decision errors to help people improve their health. *Journal of the American Medical Association, 298*(20), 2415-2417.

Loewenstein, G., and Prelec, D. (1991). Negative time preference. *American Economic Review: Papers and Proceedings, 82*(2), 347-352.

Loewenstein, G. and Prelec, D. (1993). Preferences for sequences of outcomes. *Psychological Review, 100*(1), 91-108.

Loewenstein, G., Read, D. and Baumeister, R. (Eds.). (2003). *Time and Decision: Economic and Psychological Perspectives on Intertemporal Choice.* New York: Russell Sage Foundation Press.

Loewenstein, G., and Sicherman, N. (1991). Do workers prefer increasing wage profiles? *Journal of Labor Economics, 9*, 67-84.

Lund, T., and Villadsen, E. (2005). Who retires early and why? Determinants of early retirement pension among Danish employees 57-62 years. *European Journal of Ageing, 2(4), 275-280.*

Lusardi, A., and Mitchell, O. (2007). Financial literacy and retirement preparedness: Evidence and implication for financial education. *Business Economics, 42*(1), 35-44.

Manton, K. G., Gu, X., and Lamb, V. L. (2006). Change in chronic disability from 1982-2004/2005 as measured by long-term changes in function and health in the U. S. elderly population. *Proceedings of the National Academy Sciences, 103*(48), 18374-18379.

Mather, M., and Carstensen, L. L. (2003). Aging and attentional biases for emotional faces. *Psychological Sciences, 14*, 409-415.

Mather, M., and Carstensen, L. L. (2005). Aging and motivated cognition: The positivity effect in attention and memory. *Trends in Cognitive Science, 9*(10), 496-502.

Metlife Mature Market Institute. (2007). *A profile of American Baby Boomers*. Westport, CT: Author.

Metcalfe, J., and Mischel, W. (1999). A hot/cool-system analysis of delay gratification: Dynamics of willpower. *Psychological Review, 106*(1), 3-19.

Meyer, B. J., Russo, C., and Talbot, A. (1995). Discourse comprehension and problem solving: Decisions about the treatment of breast cancer by women across the life span. *Psychology and Aging, 10*(1), 84-103.

Miller, S. M., Fang, C. Y., Manne, S. L., Engstrom, P. F., and Daly, M. B. (1999). Decision making about prophylactic oophorectomy among at-risk women: Psychological influences and implications. *Gynecological Oncology, 75*(3), 406-412.

Mischel, W., Ayduk, O., and Mendoza-Denton, R. (2003). Sustaining delay of gratification over time: A hot-cool systems perspective. In G. Loewenstein, D. Read, and R. Baumeister, (Eds.), *Time and Decision: Economic and psychological perspectives on intertemporal choice* (pp. 175-200). New York: Russell Sage.

Moser, R. P., McCaul, K., Peters, E., Nelson, W., and Marcus, S. E. (2007). Associations of perceived risk and worry with cancer health-positive actions: Data from the Health Information National Trends Survey (HINTS). *Journal of Health Psychology, 12*, 53-65.

Munnell, A. H., Golub-Sass, F., Soto, M., and Webb, A. (2008). Do households have a good sense of their retirement preparedness? *Issue in Brief 8-11*. Chestnut Hill, MA: Center for Retirement Research at Boston College.

National Center for Health Statistics. (2007). *Health, United States, 2007 with chart book on trends in the health of Americans* (Table 4; Table 22). Hyattsville, MD: U.S. Government Printing Office.

Nuttin, J. (1964). The future time perspective in human motivation and learning. *Acta Psychologica*, 23, 60-83.

Okun, M. A., and Rice, G. E. (2001). The effects of personal relevance of topic and information type on older adults' accurate recall of written medical passages about osteoarthritis. *Journal of Aging and Health, 13*(3), 410-429.

The Organisation for Economic Co-operation and Development (2001). *Aging and income: Financial resources and retirement in nine OECD countries.* Paris: Author.

Petry, N. M. (2001). Delay discounting of money and alcohol in actively using alcoholics, currently abstinent alcoholics, and controls. *Psychopharmacology, 154*, 243-250.

Petry, N. M., Bickel, W. K., and Arnett, M. (1998). Shortened time horizons and insensitivity to future consequences in heroin addicts. Addiction, 93(5), 729-738.

Read, D. and Loewenstein, D. (Eds.). (2000). Time and decision: Introduction to the special issue. *Journal of Behavioral Decision Making, 13*(2), 141-144.

Read, D., and Loewenstein, G. (1999). Enduring pain for money: Decisions based on the perceptions of memory of pain. *Journal of Behavioral Decision Making, 12*(1), 1-17.

Read, D., and Read, N. L. (2004). Time discounting over the lifespan. *Organizational Behavior and Human Decision Processes, 94*(1), 22-32.

Reynolds, B., Ortengren, A., Richards, J. B., and de Wit, H. (2006). Dimensions of impulsive behavior: Personality and behavioral measures. *Personality and Individual Differences, 40*, 305–315.

Richard, R., van der Pligt, J., and de Vries, N. (1996). Anticipated regret and time perspective: Changing sexual risk-taking behavior. *Journal of Behavioral Decision-Making, 9*(3), 185-199.

Richards, J. B., Zhang, L., Mitchell, S. H., and de Wit, H. (1999). Delay or probability discounting in a model of impulsive behavior: effect of alcohol. *Journal of the Experimental Analysis of Behavior, 71*(2), 121–143.

Rick, S., and Loewenstein, G. (2008). The role of emotion in economic behavior. In M. Lewis, J. M. Haviland-Jones, and L. F. Barrett (Eds.), *Handbook of Emotions* (3rd Ed.), (pp. 138-158). New York: The Guilford Press.

Rick, S. I., Cryder, C. E., and Loewenstein, G. (2008). Tightwads and spendthrifts. *Journal of Consumer Research, 34*(6), 767-782.

Samuelson, P. A. (1937). A Note on Measurement of Utility. *Review of Economic Studies*, 4, 155-161.

Schwartz, A., Goldberg, J., and Hazen, G. (2008). Prospect theory, reference points, and health decisions. *Judgment and Decision Making, 3*(2), 174-180.

Shultz, K.S. (2003). Bridge employment: Work after retirement. In G.A. Adams and T.A. Beehr (Eds.), *Retirement: Reasons, processes and results.* (Chapter 9, pp. 214-241). New York: Springer Publishing Company.

Social Security Administration. (2008). *A summary of the 2008 annual social security and Medicare trust fund report.* Washington, DC: Author.

Social Security Administration. (2000). *2000 Trustees Report* (Table II.F19). Washington, DC: Author.

Steinberg, L. (2008). A neurobiological perspective on adolescent risk-taking. *Developmental Review, 28*, 78-106.

Strathman, A., Gleicher, F., Boninger, D. S., and Edwards, C. S. (1994). The consideration of future consequences: Weighing immediate and distant outcomes of behavior. *Journal of Personality and Social Psychology, 66*, 742-752.

Thaler, R. (1981). Some empirical evidence on dynamic inconsistency. *Economics Letters, 8*(3), 201-207.

Trope, Y., and Liberman, N. (2003). Temporal construal. *Psychological Review, 110*, 403-421.

Trostel, P., and Taylor, G. (2001). A theory of time preference. *Economic Inquiry, 39*(3), 379-395.

Tversky, A., and Kahneman, D. (1981). The framing of decision and the psychology of choice. *Science, 211*(30), 453-458.

Tversky, A., and Kahneman, D. (1992). Advances in prospect theory: Cumulative representation of uncertainty. *Journal of Risk and Uncertainty, 5*, 297–323.

United States Administration on Aging. (2008). *A statistical profile of older Americans aged 65+*(Figure 1. Numbers of persons 65+, 1900-2030*)*. Washington, DC: Author.

United States Bureau of the Census. (2007). Minority population tops 100 million. *U.S. Census Bureau News*. Washington, D.C: U.S. Department of Commerce.

United States Department of Health and Human Services. (2002). *Physical activity fundamental to preventing disease*. Washington, DC: Author.

Van der Pol, M. M., and Cairns, J. A. (2000). Negative and zero time preference for health. *Health Economics,* 9, 171-175.

Wannamethee, S. G., Ebrahim, S., Papacosta, O., and Shaper, A. G. (2005). From a postal questionnaire of older men, healthy lifestyle factors reduced the onset of and may have increased recovery from mobility limitation. *Journal of Clinical Epidemiology, 58*(8), 831-840.

Wilson, T., and Gilbert, (2003). Affective forecasting. In M. P. Zanna (Ed.), *Advances in experimental social psychology* (vol. 35) (pp. 345-411). San Diego, CA: Elsevier Academic Press.

Zeelenberg, M. (1999). Anticipated regret, expected feedback and behavioral decision making. *Journal of Behavioral Decision-Making, 12*, 93-106.

Zeelenberg, M., van Dijk, W. W., Manstead, A. S. R., and van der Pligt, J. (1998). The experience of regret and disappointment. *Cognition and Emotion, 12*, 221-230.

Zeelenberg, M., van Dijk, W. W., Manstead, A. S. R., and van der Pligt, J. (2000). On bad decisions and disconfirmed expectancies: Regret, disappointment and decision-making. *Cognition and Emotion, 14*, 521-541.

Zwahr, M. D., Park, D. C., and Shifren, K. (1999). Judgments about estrogen replacement therapy: The role of age, cognitive abilities, and beliefs. *Psychology and Aging, 14*(2), 179-191.

In: New Directions in Aging Research
Editor: Ruby R. Brougham, pp. 167-186

ISBN 978-1-60741-976-1
© 2009 Nova Science Publishers, Inc.

Chapter 9

Goals for Retirement: Content, Structure and Process

Douglas A. Hershey*[*1] and Joy M. Jacobs-Lawson[2]
[1]Oklahoma State University, Tulsa, Oklahoma, USA
[2]University of Kentucky, Lexington, Kentucky, USA

Abstract

In this investigation the content, structure and process aspects of individuals' retirement goals were examined (cf., Austin and Vancouver, 1996). Working American adults (N = 184) aged 20 - 64 years (*M* = 41.8 yrs.) made four ratings for each of twelve commonly cited retirement goals. For each goal, individuals rated how important it was (goal importance), the amount of thought and effort they had allocated toward achieving it (goal striving), the likelihood that it actually would be achieved (goal expectancy), and how bad it would be if the goal was not met (outcome consequence). Factor analytic work revealed support for a two-factor model that distinguished self-oriented retirement goals from goals involving others. Furthermore, path analyses revealed that goal expectancy was well predicted on the basis of goal striving, among other factors. Surprisingly, age differences in individuals' goal ratings were not particularly pronounced, perhaps due to the strong social forces that serve to shape Americans' long-range retirement lifestyle aspirations. The findings from this study have clear implications for the development of future theoretical models of retirement goal-setting.

Introduction

For most individuals, the challenge of deciding upon a set of retirement goals and successfully accomplishing them is an important developmental task. Many strive to do well, but find that for one reason or another, they are unable to achieve their goals. Although

* Voice: (405) 744-4594, e-mail: douglas.hershey@okstate.edu

theoretical models of goal-setting have been prominent in the psychological literature since the early 1900s (see Locke and Latham, 1990 for a review), few empirical investigations of *retirement* goal setting have been published. In fact, a recent PsychInfo search of empirical studies using the keyword "goals" returned 4,953 hits, but when the search was constrained to the keywords "retirement" and "goals" the number of dropped to a mere 13 publications. Nine of these thirteen papers have appeared since the year 2000. Based on these findings, it would seem that research on the topic of retirement goals is among the low-hanging fruit of the goal literature.

It is not readily apparent why so few studies of retirement goals have been published. Some might suggest that it is because the goal literature is organized around particular goal dimensions, such as financial goals or happiness goals, as opposed to focusing on goals for different life stages, as is the case with goals for retirement. We would contend, however, that unlike other life stages, retirement is a period that individuals spend years planning for and thinking about from early adulthood though old age. Virtually every person who has held a job has at some point has thought about what life will be like after he or she retires. Therefore, it would seem that most individuals should have a general sense of their goals for retirement, as well as preconceived ideas about their relative level of importance. Furthermore, it's not the case that retirement goals are inherently difficult to investigate. From a methodological perspective, there is nothing intractable about studying retirement goals relative to other types of goals that have been empirically examined (e.g., career goals, interpersonal goals). Although it is true that goal choices and goal desires are dynamic and multidimensional cognitive representations (Klein, Austin and Cooper, 2008), it is also true that they are believed to be represented at the conscious level, and therefore, directly accessible through traditional means of self-report.

There are important reasons to study retirement goals as opposed to, say, goals for "late life" or "old age." As argued in Hershey, Jacobs-Lawson, and Neukam (2002), asking individuals about late life goals may conjure up images of tasks one faces at or near the end of one's life, which may be differentially associated with perceptions of frailty, loss, and decline. Retirement, in contrast, is often optimistically thought of as a stage of life marked by novel developmental tasks and opportunities, as well as the freedom to do what you please. It is a time when the "young old" can pursue new directions or focus on long-standing interests, which previously may not have been possible due to career commitments and family responsibilities. Although for most individuals "old age" is nested within retirement, we would argue that the two are not synonymous with one another, and retirement goals are a valid topic of investigation in and of themselves.

In this paper we examine the nature of individuals' retirement goals from three different perspectives: (a) their content (i.e., what are the retirement goals individuals consider to be most important?), (b) their structure (i.e., how are different retirement goals are related to one another?), and (c) the processes that underlie goal expectancy (i.e., the extent to which different goal-related constructs are predictive of one another). These dimensions of goal research—content, structure, and process—were selected as touchstones in the present study on the basis of Austin and Vancouver's (1996) paper that established a tripartite organization of the goal literature.

The remainder of this chapter is organized as follows. We begin with a review of the empirical literature on retirement goals, organized around Austin and Vancouver's ternary classificatory scheme. Next, we introduce the empirical objectives of the present investigation, and spell out a series of specific hypotheses that underlie our research questions. We then turn to a description of the methods used to collect the data, followed by the empirical results. Finally, the chapter closes with a discussion of the implications of the investigation, with a particular focus on understanding the cognitive foundations of individuals' retirement goals.

Content, Structure and Process

Austin and Vancouver (1996) drew distinctions between three types of psychological research on goals: content research focuses on describing the content of individuals' goals within particular domains, such as financial planning, leisure, health and romance. Structural research characterizes goals in terms of their interrelationships, by focusing on the properties of goals and how they are organized in relation to one another into higher-order categories. Structural investigations often involve the use of advanced statistical techniques such as factor analysis, cluster analysis, or multi-dimensional scaling, in an effort to divine the latent structure that underlies goal pursuits. Finally, process research seeks to describe how "goal processes" guide our actions and help motivate us as we strive to achieve desired states. Process investigations focus on both antecedents and consequences of goal formation and striving (Bagozzi and Dholakia, 1999), in order to better understand how goals come into being and ultimately influence our behavior. It is not uncommon for investigators to examine goals from more than one of these three dimensions, as is the case in the present investigation.

Content studies of retirement goals are relatively rare in the psychological literature. Some content investigations have focused on singular goal dimensions, such as travel goals (Staats and Pierfelice, 2003), leisure goals (Liptak, 1990), health-related goals (Lally, 2007), and financial planning (Bernheim, Forni, Gokhaale and Kotlikoff, 2002; Murray, 1998). Other content investigations have cast a broader net, by seeking to identify a wider range of goals and desires. Lapierre, Bouffard, and Bastin (1997) published a carefully conducted empirical study on late life goals that is well worth reading; however, as mentioned above, late life goals are not synonymous with retirement goals. Thus, the goals identified in their study are not directly generalizable to the retirement period. Thurnher (1974) conducted a major empirical investigation of retirement goals that revealed thirteen important dimensions (e.g., familial, material, travel, leisure). However, in most westernized societies the concept and practice of retirement has changed somewhat since the time that paper was published, potentially limiting the generalizability of her findings to present day retirees. In one recent content investigation of retirement goals (Hershey, et al., 2002), a taxonomy of retirement goals was proposed that was based on a subset of personal goals identified in the Lapierre, et al. (1997) investigation. These investigators found evidence for nine separate categories of retirement goals which included exploration, attainment of possessions, leisure, self, contact with others, contributions to others, spiritual/transcendental, financial security, and "other."

Purely structural investigations of retirement goals are absent in the psychological literature. Many older yet still highly cited (non-retirement) structural models have been published, including Murray's (1938) goal compendium, Miller, Galanter, and Pribram's (1960) cognitive formulation of goal structures, Ford and Nichols (1987) bipartite taxonomy which distinguishes within-person goals from person-environment goals, and Wicker, Lambert, Richardson and Kahler's (1984) hierarchical taxonomy of goal structures. Again, these structural representations were designed to account for interrelationships between general life goals, not goals for retirement. A more recent goal structure formulation can be seen in the work of Chulef, Read, and Walsh (2001). These authors used cluster analysis techniques to reduce 135 different major life goals gleaned from the literature into 30 distinct goal clusters. These thirty clusters were further reduced into three broad categories: (a) family, marriage, sex and romance, (b) interpersonal goals relating to interacting with people in general, and (c) intrapersonal goals. Perhaps the study of greatest relevance to the present investigation was conducted by Rapkin and Fischer (1992), who studied the goal structures of older adults (average age 73 years) using an enhanced version of the Life Goals Inventory (Bühler, Brind, and Horner, 1968). These authors found evidence that 112 different personal goals from 16 different life dimensions could be best described using a 10-factor solution. In sum, the literature on personal goal taxonomies has produced equivocal results when it comes to the identification of a common set of goal structures, or even agreement regarding the number of higher-order goals that guide our behavior. Therefore, they contribute little toward the understanding of individuals' retirement goals.

Our review of the literature revealed that more investigations have focused on process aspects of retirement goals than on content and structure studies combined. Perhaps this is due to a differential emphasis on understanding the functional aspects of goals—that is, how and why they arise, and once manifest, how they shape our behavior. The majority of work in this area has concentrated on the latter issue, that is, how clear and specific life goals influence our actions.

A series of intriguing process investigations on goal directedness have been carried out by Robbins and his colleagues at Virginia Commonwealth University. Across a series of studies among older adults, Robbins found that goal directedness (i.e., possessing stable life goals) was positively related a successful adjustment to the retirement lifestyle (Robbins, Lee and Wan, 1994; Payne, Robbins and Dougherty, 1991; Robbins, Payne and Chartrand, 1990; Smith and Robbins, 1988). Other investigations similarly found evidence pointing to the beneficial effects of having clear and specific retirement goals. Lapierre, Dubé, Bouffard and Alain (2007) found that psychologically distressed early retirees who attended a personal goal realization program showed a significant increase in hope, serenity, flexibility and a positive attitude toward retirement relative to controls (see also Lapierre, Baillargeon and Bouffard, 2001). In a somewhat older study, Rapkin and Fischer (1992) found that older adults who possessed energetic life-style goals demonstrated higher levels of life satisfaction. Although the "lifestyle goals" measured in this study were not retirement goals *per se*, all 179 participants in the investigation were retired at the time of testing. A small number of studies have revealed that the nature of workers' personal goals serve as good predictors of departure from the workforce (e.g., Brougham and Walsh, 2005, 2007; Adams, 1999). Finally, in a community-based intervention study, Hershey, Mowen, and Jacobs-Lawson (2003) found that retirement goal-setting exercises served to facilitate engagement in pre-retirement planning activities.

In three different process investigations of financial planning for retirement carried out by Hershey and his colleagues (Hershey, Henkens and van Dalen, 2007; Hershey, Jacobs-Lawson, McArdle and Hamagami, 2007; Stawski, Hershey and Jacobs-Lawson, 2007), one's level of retirement goal clarity was found to be an excellent predictor of not only financial knowledge acquisition, but also the enactment of pre-retirement financial planning tasks. Furthermore, Jacobs-Lawson (2003) demonstrated that retirement goal clarity covaried with age in adulthood (older adults had clearer goals than their younger counterparts), and goal clarity was related to the perceived importance of the characteristics of various retirement saving investments. Taken together, the effects witnessed in process studies provide compelling evidence that retirement goals, when held in a clear and specific form, have an unequivocally beneficial impact on future development and psychological well-being.

In the following section of the paper, we describe how retirement goals are examined in the present investigation.

Present Study

This study is an extension of the Hershey, et al. (2002) content investigation of pre-retirees' goals for retirement. In that investigation, researchers examined the frequency with which different retirement goals were cited during the course a semi-structured interview. This study is also a content study, in part, in which we take a step in a more parametrically-oriented direction. Specifically, participants made importance ratings for twelve personal goal dimensions often cited as being associated with retirement. We selected these goals on the basis of overlap seen across four goal studies focusing on retirement and late life (Chulef, et al., 2001; Hershey, et al, 2002; Lapierre, et al., 1997; Rapkin and Fisher, 1992).

Analysis of goal importance ratings—just one of the types of ratings collected in this investigation—is a technique researchers often use to identify the meaningfulness of individuals' personal goals. One of the more modest (but nonetheless significant) objectives of this study was descriptive in nature—to get a clear sense of which of the twelve goals are considered to be most important, and which ones are considered least important.

A second objective was to examine the structural basis of the twelve retirement goals; that is, the extent to which they are related to one another. As pointed out in the literature review, factor analysis is often the statistical technique of choice in structural studies of this type. This study was no different, as we subjected the retirement goal data to exploratory factor analysis. What set this investigation apart, however, is the type of personal goals we examined—that is, those specific to retirement. Also, unique about this study was the fact that our analyses are based on a relatively small number of high-level personal goal dimensions drawn from the existing psychological literature. Therefore, in contrast to other studies that identify a large number of factors (perhaps 10 or more) based on sometimes dozens of indicators, we anticipated that only a small number of "meta-level" goals (cf., Kuhn, 2005) would be identified—that is, if an interpretable solution could be found.

The third empirical objective was to examine the process relations between four different retirement goal constructs. In addition to measuring goal importance for the twelve retirement goals, we asked participants to rate: (a) how bad it would be if a particular goal was not achieved (outcome consequence), (b) how much thought and effort they put into achieving the goal (goal striving), and (c) the likelihood that they would actually achieve the goal (goal expectancy). These four variables were tested alongside one another in the path analysis model depicted in Figure 1. The constructs in the model were ordered based on the following assumptions. First, it was hypothesized that perceptions of "how bad" it would be if a goal were not achieved would determine individuals' perceptions of goal importance (Ajzen and Fishbein, 1980, 2005; Fishbein and Ajzen, 1975). Second, it was predicted that the perceived importance of a goal would be positively related to the amount of thought and effort one allocates toward achieving a goal (Beach, 1998; Beach and Mitchell, 1987). And third, it was expected that the amount of thought and effort one allocates to achieving a goal should be positively related to goal expectancy (Weiner and Graham, 1999). In addition to testing these three direct paths connecting adjacent variables (paths *a, b,* and *c*), three additional (indirect) paths were tested (paths *d, e,* and *f*), thereby forming the basis of a partial mediation model.

In addition to a broad-based examination of the content, structure, and process aspects of individuals' retirement goals, these three aspects of the goal construct will be tested for age effects. As argued by Sanderson and Cantor (1999; see also Cantor and Zirkel, 1990; Nurmi, 1992; Winell, 1987), different life stages are marked by different life tasks, goals, strategies and outcomes. Therefore, it is not inconceivable that younger and older study participants might hold differing ideas about the importance of different retirement goals, how they are structured relative to one another, and how they influence behavior.

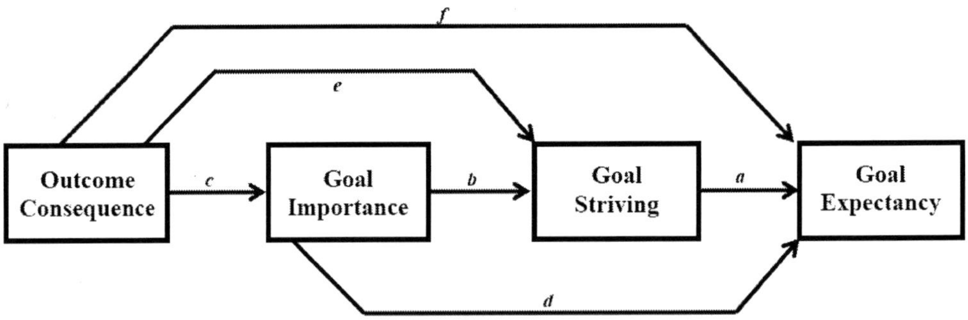

Figure 1. Representation of the path model used to examine the process aspects of individuals' retirement goal dimensions. In this partial mediation model, which was tested separately for all twelve goals, both direct and indirect paths were estimated.

Method

Participants

A total of 189 working pre-retirees (94 women; 95 men) served as voluntary participants in the study. The sample ranged in age from 20 – 64 years (M = 41.76, SD = 12.73). At the time of testing a large majority of participants were employed on a full-time basis (82%), the remaining individuals (18%) were employed on a part-time basis, and none reported having ever been previously retired. Participants had completed on average 14.99 years of education (*SD* = 2.14), had a median household income of $50,000, and somewhat over half of respondents (59%) were married. For some of the analyses we describe, the sample is subdivided into two age groups each spanning 22 years: younger adults ($n = 93$; aged 20 - 42) and older adults ($n = 91$; aged 43 - 65).

Procedure

Participation in the study was solicited at public locations in North Central Oklahoma (e.g., recreation areas, community centers, businesses, shopping centers). An effort was made to sample equivalent numbers of men and women whose age range covered the traditional working lifespan. Participants were prescreened to ensure that they met the inclusionary criteria for the study, which was that they be employed on at least a half-time basis (20 hours/week), and report not having previously been retired. Questionnaires were completed individually or in small groups of 2-4 persons.

Materials

Respondents' primary task was to rate each of twelve different retirement goals along four dimensions: (a) the importance of the goal (hereafter, goal importance), (b) how much thought and effort had been put into achieving the goal (goal striving), (c) how likely it is that the goal will be achieved (goal expectancy), and (d) how bad it would be if the goal was *not* achieved (outcome consequence). All ratings were made using a 7-point unidirectional response scale. Anchor terms for the importance dimension were 1 = *not at all important,* 7 = *extremely important;* for the goal striving dimension 1 = *little or no thought/effort,* 7 = *a great deal of thought/effort;* for the goal expectancy dimension 1 = *extremely unlikely,* 7 = *extremely likely*; and for the outcome consequence dimension 1 = *not bad at all,* 7 = *extremely horrible.*

The twelve goals selected for inclusion in this investigation were: (a) spending time with family members (FAMILY), (b) pursuing a specific hobby or hobbies (HOBBIES), (c) participating in volunteer activities or helping others (VOLUNTEER), (d) being financially stable and independent (FINANCIAL), (e) being healthy and physically fit (HEALTH), (e) being happy and enjoying life (HAPPY), (f) being a wise person (WISDOM), (g) being relaxed (RELAXING), (h) experiencing a high quality of life (HIGH QUALITY LIFE), (i) spiritual or religious activities (SPIRITUALITY), (j) spending time with friends or other retirees (FRIENDS), and (k) travel (TRAVEL). To establish a consistent goal "frame," all goals were portrayed using a positive valence (cf., Winell, 1987)—for instance, "being healthy and physically fit" as opposed to "avoiding health problems and physical decline."

Results

In this section of the paper, we present findings from the content, structural and process analyses, in that order. All members of the sample were treated as a single group in these three sets of analyses. In the final section of the results, we turn our attention to age differences in the content, structure and process aspects of individuals' retirement goals. This is accomplished by subdividing the sample into two separate age groups.

Content Analysis of Ratings

We begin our analysis by presenting summary data from the importance ratings for the various retirement goal dimensions. Figure 2 shows a bar graph that lists each of the twelve retirement goals, arranged in descending order of mean level of importance. Across all respondents, the most important goal was to "be happy" in retirement, with an average score that nearly topped the 7-unit response scale. The desire for happiness was closely followed by the goals of being financially secure, enjoying good health, and having time to spend with family members.

The least important goals included travel and participating in volunteer activities, which were rated fully two points (on average) lower than the most highly rated goal dimensions. This score differential suggests a fair amount of variability in terms of relative levels of perceived importance. It is worth noting, however, that the means for travel and volunteering were still to the right of the midpoint on the scale, which indicates that even these goals were considered to be moderately important.

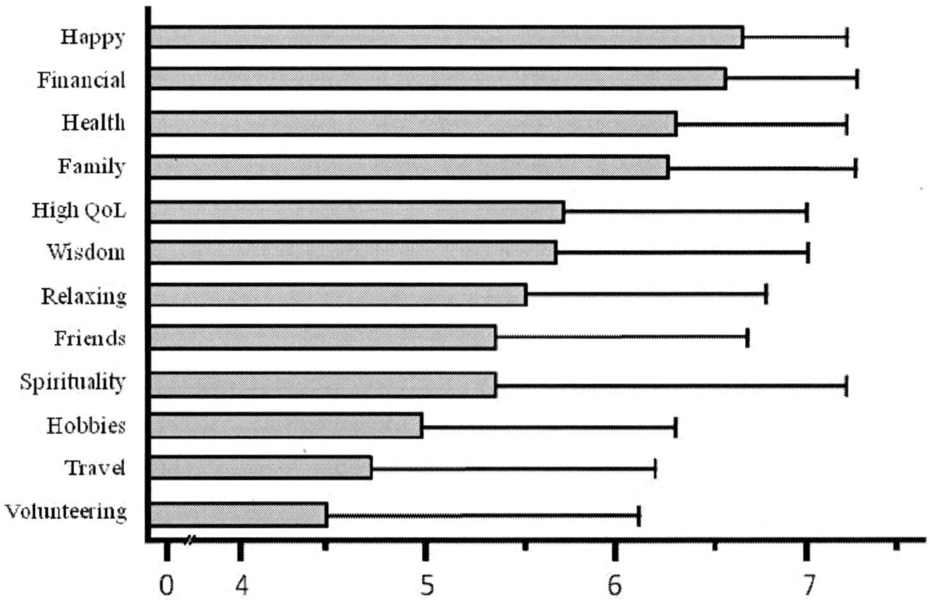

Figure 2. Bar graph of mean importance ratings (and standard deviations) for the twelve retirement goal dimensions.

Table 1. Mean Ratings for Goal Striving, Goal Expectancy, and Outcome Consequence

	Goal Striving		Goal Expectancy		Outcome Consequence	
Retirement Goal	Mean	(*SD*)	Mean	(*SD*)	Mean	(*SD*)
Happy	5.96	(1.33)	6.14	(0.91)	5.86	(1.40)
Financial	5.81	(1.28)	5.74	(1.07)	5.60	(1.49)
Health	5.40	(1.40)	5.44	(1.07)	5.52	(1.43)
Family	5.41	(1.64)	6.11	(1.11)	5.60	(1.54)
High QoL	5.16	(1.55)	5.46	(1.26)	4.96	(1.60)
Wisdom	4.92	(1.59)	5.23	(1.30)	4.61	(1.59)
Relaxing	4.76	(1.62)	5.27	(1.27)	4.49	(1.55)
Friends	4.70	(1.66)	5.19	(1.34)	4.60	(1.71)
Spirituality	4.95	(1.96)	5.40	(1.72)	4.94	(1.99)
Hobbies	4.30	(1.63)	5.15	(1.39)	3.81	(1.62)
Travel	4.00	(1.70)	5.05	(1.46)	3.35	(1.65)
Volunteering	3.77	(1.66)	4.64	(1.59)	3.68	(1.65)

Note: Goals are ordered in descending order of mean importance ratings.

Another intriguing aspect of the importance ratings was the increase in variability seen as a function of decreases in mean scores. In short, there was greater score agreement across participants surrounding the more highly rated goals (e.g., be happy, financial security) than the goals that earned lower mean ratings (e.g., volunteer activities, spirituality/religion).

In addition to the goal importance ratings described above, mean scores and standard deviations were calculated for ratings of goal striving, goal expectancy and outcome consequence. These three sets of scores are shown in Table 1. Visual inspection of the table reveals a high degree of convergence between the importance ratings found in Figure 2 and these three related goal dimensions. More will be said about the inter-relationships between the goal importance ratings and these additional three sets of scores in the process analyses described below.

Structure of the Goal Dimensions

Exploratory factor analyses were computed to examine the latent structure of the twelve goals. The factor analysis graphically diagrammed in Figure 3 is based on a principle components analysis extraction followed by promax rotation to a final solution. The first factor—which represents the self-oriented retirement goals—had an eigenvalue of 2.50 and accounted for 20.9 percent of the total variance. This factor had six positive loadings greater than 0.45: financial stability, good health, happiness, wisdom, relaxation, and a high quality of life.

The second factor—which represents retirement goals involving others—had an eigenvalue of 1.93 and accounted for 16.1 percent of the total variance. The four items with appreciable loadings on this factor included: spending time with family members, volunteering/helping others, spiritual and religious activities, and spending time with friends. Two items—travel and the pursuit of hobbies—failed to reveal appreciable loadings on either factor and therefore, is not shown in Figure 3. Together, the two factors accounted for 36.44 percent of the variance in the model.

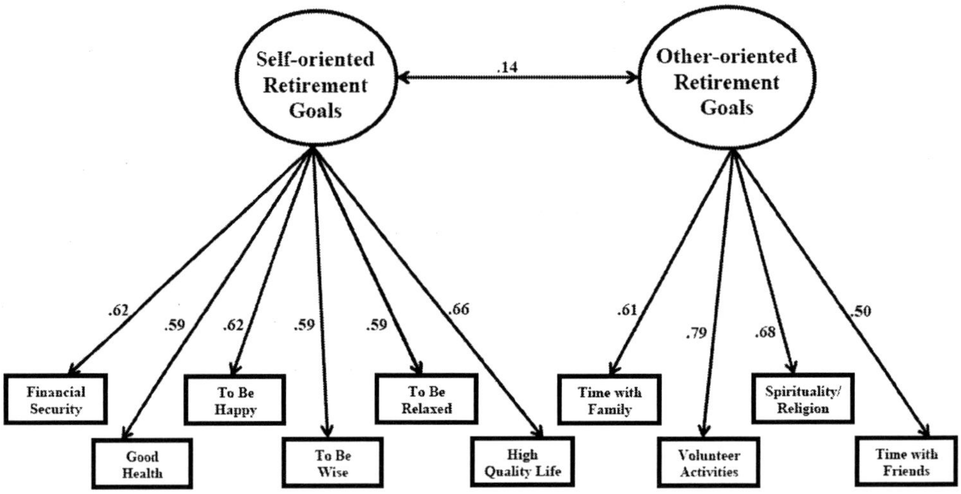

Figure 3. Two-factor structure for the retirement goal dimensions. The pattern of loadings reveals the existence of six self-oriented and four other-oriented retirement goals (two factors with loadings of less than .45 have been omitted for clarity).

A promax rotation method was specifically selected for this analysis to examine the possibility of the two factors being correlated with one another; however, the factor correlation matrix failed to indicate this was the case. As seen in the figure, the observed correlation between the self- and other-related factors was only $r = .14$.

As a follow-up to the structural analysis, mean importance scores were calculated for the self- and other-oriented goal dimensions. For the six self-oriented goals, the average score was found to be 6.07 (*SD* = 0.65). For the four other-oriented goals, the mean importance rating was 5.35 (SD = 0.99), which is a statistically reliable difference, $t(188) = 9.12, p < .01$.

Process Aspects of the Retirement Goals

A series of hierarchical regressions were conducted in order to examine the processes that underlie perceptions of goal expectancy (i.e., the perceived likelihood the goal will be achieved). Toward this end, twelve separate path analysis models were tested, one for each goal dimension, the general form of which is diagrammed in Figure 1. As seen in the figure, the model contains three direct paths (*a, b* and *c*) and three indirect paths (*d, e* and *f*). The outcomes for these analyses are summarized in Table 2, including standardized beta weights for each significant path and adjusted *R*-squared values for each endogenous variable in the path model.

Looking first at the adjusted *R*-squared values for goal expectancy, the differences in variance accounted for across goal dimensions is striking. For the volunteering and spirituality dimensions, over 60 percent of the variability in goal expectancy was captured.

Only about half that amount of variance, in contrast, was explained among the finances and family dimensions.

Table 2. Standardized Beta Weights and R-squared Values from the Path Analyses Designed to Examine Process Aspects of Retirement Goal Dimensions

Path	Financial	Health	Happy	Wisdom	Relaxing	High QoL
Direct Paths						
a: Goal Striving →Goal expectancy	.53**	.66**	.56**	.63**	.58**	.55**
b: Goal Importance →Goal Striving	.32**	.23**	.57**	.66*	.60**	.70**
c: Outcome Consequence →Goal Importance	.51**	.47**	.27**	.61**	.49**	.63**
Indirect Paths						
d: Goal Importance →Goal expectancy	.14*	.52**	.21**	.40**	.49**	.31**
e: Outcome Consequence →Goal Striving	.20*	.19**	--	.24**	.16*	.16*
f: Outcome Consequence →Goal expectancy	--	--	--	.17*	--	.17*
Explained Variance						
R2 Goal expectancy	.29	.47	.33	.49	.48	.35
R2 Goal Striving	.12	.29	.32	.46	.38	.51
R2 Goal Importance	.26	.22	.07	.37	.24	.40

Path	Family	Volunteer	Spirituality	Friends	Travel	Hobbies
Direct Paths						
a: Goal Striving →Goal expectancy	.49**	.68**	.78**	.65**	.59**	.59**
b: Goal Importance →Goal Striving	.56**	.74**	.86**	.67**	.52**	.65**
c: Outcome Consequence →Goal Importance	.51**	.69**	.77**	.62**	.57**	.60**
Indirect Paths						
d: Goal Importance →Goal expectancy	.16*	.48**	.37**	.35**	.28**	.47**
e: Outcome Consequence →Goal Striving	--	--	--	.27**	.26**	--

Table 2. (Continued)

Path	Family	Volunteer	Spirituality	Friends	Travel	Hobbies
f: Outcome Consequence →Goal expectancy	.21**	.37**	.25**	.24**	.14*	--
Explained Variance						
R2 Goal expectancy	.27	.63	.66	.52	.42	.47
R2 Goal Striving	.31	.55	.73	.49	.31	.43
R2 Goal Importance	.26	.47	.59	.38	.33	.35

* $p < .05$; ** $p < .01$.

Note: For each analysis (shown in separate columns), beta weight entries correspond to the paths shown in figure two. A dash indicates a nonsignificant coefficient.

Virtually all goal dimensions revealed strong positive relationships between the reported level of goal striving and perceptions of goal expectancy (i.e., path *a*). In fact, across the twelve dimensions, the average standardized beta weight for this path was .61. What seemed to distinguish models with large amounts of explained variance for goal expectancy from those that were less predictive was the impact of the indirect paths (i.e., paths *d* and *f*). The effect of these two paths was appreciable for the volunteering and spirituality dimensions, whereas it was either small or non-existent for goal dimensions such as family, finances, and happiness.

Overall, less variance was accounted for when it came to the goal striving and goal importance constructs. This could be due, in part, to the reduced number of indicators in the model relative to the expectancy construct. Notably, the dimensions that showed the most explained variance for the goal striving and goal importance scores—volunteering and spirituality—were the same dimensions that captured the most variance in the goal expectancy analysis.

In addition to the twelve dimension-specific process models described above, two other process models were calculated—one for the combined set of self-oriented goals (based on the six previously identified goal dimensions in the structural analysis), and a second for the combined set of other-oriented goals (which was based on the four previously identified dimensions). As seen in table 3, an appreciable amount of variance in goal expectancy was captured for both of these dimensions (.60 versus .50, respectively). Also notable was the difference across analyses in the amount of explained variance for the goal striving and goal importance constructs. Specifically, the adjusted *R*-squared values for the other-oriented analysis were substantially higher than the self-oriented analysis, which suggests that more systematic variance was operating in the former. As was the case in the analyses for the twelve individual goal dimensions shown in Table 2, for the two computations shown in Table 3 all three direct paths revealed extremely strong effects, with more modest predictive contributions stemming from the indirect influences.

Table 3. Standardized Beta Weights and R-squared Values from the Path Analyses Examining Self-Oriented and Other-Oriented Goals

Path	Self	Others
Direct Paths		
a: Goal Striving→Goal expectancy	.67**	.69**
b: Goal Importance→Goal Striving	.60**	.73**
c: Outcome Consequence→Goal Importance	.54**	.68**
Indirect Paths		
d: Goal Importance→Goal expectancy	.29**	.39**
e: Outcome Consequence→Goal Striving	--	--
f: Outcome Consequence→Goal expectancy	--	.29**
Explained Variance		
R2 Goal expectancy	.50	.60
R2 Goal Striving	.35	.52
R2 Goal Importance	.29	.46

** $p < .01$.

Age Differences in Retirement Goals

Based on the theoretical possibility that the nature of individuals' retirement goals differ at various points in the adulthood, we carried out analyses to test for the influence of age on goal content, structure, and process. In terms of the content analyses, mean score comparisons were carried out (accompanied by analysis-wise Bonferonni adjustments) to test for age differences in importance ratings. Only one of the twelve goal dimensions—"being in good health"—revealed a reliable difference across groups. Specifically, older adults' health ratings ($M = 6.54$, $SD = 0.67$) were significantly larger than those of younger respondents ($M = 6.15$, $SD = 0.95$), $t(187) = 3.32$, $p = .01$. Beyond that effect, the rank orders of the perceived importance ratings across age groups were nearly identical. The four most important goals for younger individuals included finances, happiness, time spent with family, and good health (in descending order of importance), whereas they were happiness, good health, finances, and time spent with family for the older members of the sample. The least important goals for younger individuals were hobbies, travel and volunteering; the same three goals appeared at the bottom of the list for older individuals in a somewhat different order. In sum, few noteworthy differences emerged in the age-based content ratings for the specific dimensions.

In addition to examining age differences in importance ratings, we probed for evidence of developmental effects among the other three goal-related constructs—outcome consequence, expectancy, and goal striving—at the level of self- and other-oriented goals. No age differences in self and other goals were identified for the former two constructs, however, the goal striving construct did reveal age differences. Specifically, self-oriented goal striving scores were higher for older adults ($M = 5.55$, $SD = 0.86$) than younger participants ($M = 5.12$, $SD = 1.16$), $t(187) = 2.51$, $p < .01$; and other-oriented goal striving scores were also higher for older adults ($M = 4.97$, $SD = 1.06$) relative to their younger counterparts ($M = 4.45$, $SD = 1.32$), $t(187) = 2.95$, $p < .01$.

In terms of developmental differences, the analysis of the two-factor retirement goal structure using importance ratings was also quite interesting. Two separate principle component analyses (one for each age group) were computed in which two factors were forced, followed in each case by promax rotation to a final solution. The basic two factor (self-oriented; other-oriented) goal structure was empirically supported, but differences among age groups did emerge. Table 4 shows the rotated factor loadings (greater than .45) for the two sets of goals, presented as a function of age group status. As seen in the table, the basic factor structure was similar for the two age groups. In terms of differences, the goal of "travel" was found to load on self-oriented goals for younger individuals, but on the other-oriented goal factor for older individuals.

Moreover, "being wise" revealed moderate cross-loadings among members of the young group, whereas relaxation was found to produce moderate cross-loading for older respondents. "Pursuit of hobbies" failed to produce appreciable loadings in either the young or the old model (and therefore, is not shown in the table). Finally, a notable age difference was identified in the magnitude of the factor correlations, with an association of $r = .06$ found for members of the young group, and $r = .23$ for older individuals, which indicates a stronger perceived overlap among indicators for those individuals who are nearer to retirement.

Table 4. Rotated Factor Loadings for Self- and Other-related Retirement Goals Shown as a Function of Age Group

Younger Respondents		Older Respondents	
Self Goals	Other Goals	Self Goals	Other Goals
.54 Travel	.69 Family	.63 Financial	.58 Travel
.61 Financial	.77 Volunteer	.73 Health	.54 Family
.51 Health	.52 Wisdom	.54 Happy	.77 Volunteer
.58 Happy	.70 Spirituality	.71 Wisdom	.56 Relaxing
.48 Wisdom	.52 Friends	.55 Relaxing	.50 Spirituality
.63 Relaxing		.73 High QoL	.42 Friends
.63 High QoL			

Note: Goals with loadings less than .45 have been omitted for clarity.

The possibility of age effects in the process model (see Figure 1) was also considered. Toward this end, 24 separate path analysis models were calculated using hierarchical regression; that is, one model for each age group for each of the twelve goal dimensions. Looking across the 24 models, no clear cut pattern of age effects was apparent. Age differences in *R*-squared values and beta weights were identified, but not in a consistent manner across multiple retirement goal dimensions, thus making it difficult to draw any general age-related conclusions. Overall, these analyses indicate that the process aspects of these four goal dimensions—that is, associations between outcome consequence, importance, striving, and goal expectancy—are relatively age invariant.

In an effort to be thorough, four other process analyses were conducted—two models (one for each age group) for self-oriented goals, and two additional models (one for each age group) for other-oriented goals. For this analysis, mean self and other scores were calculated for the various constructs (striving, importance, expectancy, outcome consequence). Table 5 presents the results from these four process models. As was the case for the self/other models for the entire sample, in these analyses more variance was explained for the other-oriented goal constructs compared to the self-oriented goals. Also apparent from a visual inspection of the table is the fact that relative to the other-oriented goals, age differences were more pronounced in the self-oriented models. In fact, twice as much variance was explained for goal importance in the young self model (R^2 = .40) than the old self model (R^2 = .19), and a similar age effect was witnessed for the other-oriented analyses (.53 versus .37). A reversal in the direction of this age effect was identified for goal striving, with more of the variance captured among older individuals (46 percent) compared to younger participants (30 percent).

Table 5. Standardized Beta Weights and R-squared Values for the Process Models Designed to Examine Age (Young; Old) and Goal Type (Self; Other)

Path	Young Self	Old Self	Young Other	Old Other
Direct Paths				
a: Goal Striving →Goal expectancy	.65**	.72**	.69**	.72**
b: Goal Importance →Goal Striving	.55**	.69**	.70**	.80**
c: Outcome Consequence →Goal Importance	.64**	.44**	.73**	.61**
Indirect Paths				
d: Goal Importance →Goal expectancy	.33*	--	.36**	.41**
e: Outcome Consequence →Goal Striving	--	--	--	--
f: Outcome Consequence →Goal expectancy	--	--	.30**	.29**
Explained Variance				
R2 Goal expectancy	.49	.51	.56	.63
R2 Goal Striving	.30	.46	.50	.63
R2 Goal Importance	.40	.19	.53	.37

* $p < .05$; ** $p < .01$.

Discussion

The results of this study reinforce previous goal-related empirical findings, and at the same time, contribute new insights into workers' aspirations for retirement. It was no surprise that the goals selected for inclusion in this investigation were all perceived to be, at the very least, moderately important (in fact, four of the twelve goals were rated as *extremely* important). One reason for this is because the goals individuals rated had, in previous investigations, been identified as highly valued. Furthermore, the factor analytic work revealed that the set of retirement goals had a clearly interpretable dual factor structure, which is a novel empirical contribution to this narrow area of the literature on goals. Finally, the process model that was tested helped to paint a clearer picture of the way retirement goals arise, and how they influence both behavior and cognitions.

With regard to the content of individuals' retirement goals, it was somewhat surprising to see just how highly individuals rated the importance of being happy, financial independence, good health, and time spent with family members. Not only were the mean ratings for these dimensions quite near the top of the rating scale, but they were also accompanied by extremely low standard errors, which suggests that they possess a high degree of universal appeal. This near-universal agreement was unexpected in light of the divergent set of trajectories individuals take on the path to retirement and old age (Dannefer, 1988; Frazier, Newman and Jaccard, 2007; van Solinge, 2006). One issue that is not clear from the analysis of the content data is whether the same behavioral pursuits sufficient to make one happy in midlife, for example, are comparable to the ones sufficient to make a person happy during retirement. That is, without knowledge of the specific micro-behaviors that underlie retirement happiness, it is not possible to draw definitive conclusions about the precursors to happiness at different points in the life span. Specific goals may reflect apples at one point in a person's life and oranges at a different life stage, but they would all be identified as fruits (or in the present case, happiness) when examined using global importance score ratings.

The structural analyses produced interesting findings as well. It would appear on the basis of previous research that retirement goals are, in some respects, comparable to personal goals held at other points in the life span. That is, the two-factor (self/other) structure identified in this investigation fits well with the bipartite structure of within-person goals and person/environment goals identified by Ford and Nichols (1987; see also Winell, 1987 on this distinction). Small age differences in these goal structures, however, indicate that the perceived organization of retirement goals is *not* developmentally invariant. In order to probe the limits of age invariance, future studies might focus on age differences in retirement goal structures cross-culturally. Particularly valuable would be investigations that utilize societies or cultural sub-groups in which there exists appreciable variability in age-graded behavioral norms (Cantor and Zirkel, 1990) or tasks (Nurmi, 1992).

The process analyses revealed conflicting findings. On the one hand, the path analysis findings reported in Table 2 for the twelve goal dimensions suggest that the theoretical model shown in Figure 1 is not conceptually unreasonable. On the other hand, the large observed discrepancies in slopes and R-squared values across models suggest that the mechanisms that underlie goal expectancy differ, to some extent, on the basis of the specific domain being considered.

It is interesting to speculate how much within-person developmental variability exists among the set of hypothesized relationships in the process models, despite the absence of clear-cut age effects reported in the results section above. We acknowledge that the process model tested in Figure 1 represents a snapshot of individuals' higher-level goals at a single point in time, but actual goal behaviors (and the processes that underlie them) might be expected to shift dynamically over time (Klein, et al., 2008). How do one's perceptions of outcome consequence and goal importance change as a function of changes in perceptions of goal expectancy? That is, in the face of evidence that we may not achieve a particular goal, do we readily discount the consequence of goal failure, and accordingly, psychologically reduce its perceived importance? Or, do individuals stubbornly cling to their goal-attainment convictions despite the fact that our goals may ultimately be unattainable? A deeper understanding of retirement goal processes from an age-graded cybernetic perspective would be of value (Locke and Latham, 2006), particularly in light of the way individuals' behavioral needs, interests and desires shift over the course of the life span.

This study is potentially limited by the fact that a self-report measure of goal striving was employed, which may have resulted in a selective reporting bias. Perhaps future studies could use more objective indicators of goal striving (e.g., amount of income saved; research on travel destinations; concrete plans for hobbies) in an effort to enhance measurement sensitivity for this construct. A second factor that limits the generalizability of the findings involves the fact that respondents were sampled from one state, and their household income was somewhat higher than the national average. This could have resulted in a skewed representation of the nature of individuals' retirement goals. Future investigations that examine the diversity of goals among members of different racial and ethnic groups are warranted; particularly in light of the different types of work and retirement experiences they encounter (Fried and Mehrotra, 1998). Finally, the cross-sectional design of this study allowed us to test for age differences, but such a design fails to reveal pertinent information about how retirement goals *change* with age. A suitably designed longitudinal study would need to be carried out to address this important issue of age-related change.

Conclusion

In conclusion, the results of this investigation reveal that goals for retirement are in many respects similar to the personal goals individuals hold at other points in adulthood. Perhaps the small to non-existent age effects identified in the content and process aspects of retirement goals should not have come as a surprise, given that we live in a culture that indoctrinates individuals to begin thinking about retirement at an early age. As pointed out by sociologist David Ekerdt (2004), Americans are "born to retire," which is to say that our expectations and planning behaviors are shaped over a period of decades to help ensure a smooth and successful transition out of the workforce. Consistent with this perspective, stability and continuity of high-level retirement goals over the life span appears to be the rule, rather than the exception.

References

Adams, G. A. (1999). Career-related variables and planned retirement age: An extension of Beehr's model. *Journal of Vocational Behavior, 55,* 221-235.

Ajzen, I., and Fishbein, M. (1980). *Understanding attitudes and predicting social behavior.* Englewood Cliffs, NJ: Prentice-Hall.

Ajzen, I., and Fishbein, M. (2005). The influence of attitudes on behavior. In D. Albarracín, B. T. Johnson, and M. P. Zanna (Eds.), *The handbook of attitudes* (pp. 173-221). Mahwah, NJ: Erlbaum.

Austin, J. T. and Vancouver, J. B. (1996). Goal constructs in psychology: Structure, process, and content. *Psychological Bulletin, 120,* 338-375.

Bagozzi, R. P., and Dholakia, U. (1999). Goal setting and goal striving in consumer behavior. *Journal of Marketing, 63,* 19-32.

Beach, L. R. (1998). *Image theory: Theoretical and empirical foundations.* Mahwah, NJ: Erlbaum.

Beach, L. R., and Mitchell, T. R. (1987). Image theory: Principles, goals and plans in decision-making. *Acta Psychologia, 66,* 201-220.

Bernheim, B. D., Forni, L., Gokhale, J., and Kotlikoff, L. J. (2002). An economic approach to setting retirement saving goals. In O. Mitchell, Z. Bodie, B. Hammond, and S. Zeldes (Eds.), *Innovations in financing retirement* (pp. 77-105). Philadelphia: University of Pennsylvania Press.

Brougham, R. R., and Walsh, D. A. (2005). Goal expectations as predictors of retirement intentions. *International Journal of Aging and Human Development, 61,* 141-160.

Brougham, R. R., and Walsh, D. A. (2007). Image theory, goal incompatibility, and retirement intent. *International Journal of Aging and Human Development, 65,* 203-229.

Bühler, C., Brind, A., and Horner, A. (1968). Old age as a phase of human life. *Human Development, 11,* 53-63.

Cantor, N., and Zirkel, S. (1990). Personality, cognition, and purposive behavior. In L. A. Pervin (Ed.), *Handbook of personality: Theory and research* (pp. 135-164). New York: Guilford Press.

Chulef, A. S., Read, S. J., and Walsh, D. A. (2001). A hierarchical taxonomy of human goals. *Motivation and Emotion, 25,* 191-232.

Dannefer, D. (1988). What's in a name?: An account of the neglect of variability in the study of aging. In J. E. Birren and V. L. Bengtson (Eds.) *Emergent theories of aging* (pp. 356-384). New York, Springer.

Ekerdt, D. J. (2004). Born to retire: The foreshortened life course. *The Gerontologist, 44,* 3-9.

Fishbein, M., and Ajzen, I. (1975). *Belief, attitude, intention, and behavior: An introduction to theory and research.* Reading, MA: Addison-Wesley.

Ford, M. E., and Nichols, C. W. (1987). A taxonomy of human goals and some possible applications. In M. E. Ford and D. H. Ford (Eds.), *Humans as self-constructing systems: Putting the framework to work* (pp. 289-311). Hillsdale, NJ: Erlbaum.

Frazier, L. D., Newman, F. L., and Jaccard, J. (2007). Psychosocial outcomes in later life: A multivariate model. *Psychology and Aging, 22,* 676-689.

Fried, S. B., and Mehrotra, C. M. (1998). *Aging and diversity: An active learning experience.* New York: Taylor and Francis.

Hershey, D. A., Henkens, K., and Van Dalen, H. P. (2007). Mapping the minds of retirement planners. *Journal of Cross-Cultural Psychology, 38*(3), 361-382.

Hershey, D. A., Jacobs-Laweson, J. M., McArdle, J. J., and Hamagami, F. (2007). Psychological foundation of financial planning for retirement. *Journal of Adult Development, 14*(1-2), 26-36.

Hershey, D. A., Jacobs-Lawson, J. M., and Neukam, K. A. (2002). Influences of age and gender on workers' goals for retirement. *International Journal of Aging and Human Development, 55,* 163-179.

Hershey, D. A., Mowen, J. C., and Jacobs-Lawson, J. M. (2003). An experimental comparison of retirement planning intervention seminars. *Educational Gerontology, 29,* 339-359.

Jacobs-Lawson, J. M. (2003). Influences of age and investor characteristics on women's retirement investment decisions (Doctoral dissertation, Oklahoma State University, 2003). *Dissertation Abstracts International: Section B, 64,* 9B.

Klein, H. K., Austin, J. T., and Cooper, J. T. (2008). Goal choice and decision processes. In R. Kanfer, G. Chen, and R. Pritchard (Eds.), *Work motivation: Past, present, and future* (pp 101-150). Abingdon, England: Routledge Academic.

Kuhn, D. (2005). *Education for thinking.* Cambridge, MA: Harvard University Press.

Lally, P. (2007). Identity and athletic retirement: A prospective study. *Psychology of Sport and Exercise, 8,* 85-99.

Lapierre, S., Baillargeon, J., and Bouffard, L. (2001). Tenacity and flexibility in the pursuit of personal goals: Impact of retirement and well-being. *Canadian Journal on Aging, 20,* 557-576.

Lapierre, S., Bouffard, L., and Bastin, E. (1997). Personal goals and subjective well-being in later life. *International Journal of Aging and Human Development, 45,* 287-303.

Lapierre, S., Dubé, M., Bouffard, L., and Alain, M. (2007). Addressing suicidal ideations through the realization of meaningful personal goals. *Crisis: The Journal of Crisis Intervention and Suicide Prevention, 28,* 16-25.

Liptak, J. J. (1990). Preretirement counseling: Integrating the leisure planning component. *Career Development Quarterly, 38,* 360-367.

Locke, E. A., and Latham, G. P. (1990). *A theory of goal-setting and task performance.* Englewood Cliffs, NJ: Prentice Hall.

Miller, G. A., Galanter, E., and Pribram, K. H. (1960). *Plans and the structure of behavior.* New York: Holt.

Murray, H. C. (1938). *Explorations in personality.* New York: Oxford University Press.

Murray, M. C. (1998). More people saving, but few have goals. *National Underwriter Life and Health-Financial Services Edition, 102,* 49.

Nurmi, J. E. (1992). Age differences in adult life goals, concerns, and their temporal extension: A life course approach to future –oriented motivation. *International Journal of Behavioral Development, 15,* 487-508.

Payne, E. C., Robbins, S. B., and Dougherty, L. (1991). Goal directedness and older-adult adjustment. *Journal of Counseling Psychology, 38,* 302-308.

Rapkin, B. D., and Fischer, K. (1992). Personal goals of older adults: Issues in assessment and prediction. *Psychology and Aging, 7,* 127-137.

Robbins, S. B., Lee, R. M., and Wan, T. T. H. (1994). Goal continuity as a mediator of early retirement adjustment: Testing a multidimensional model. *Journal of Counseling Psychology, 41,* 18-26.

Robbins, S. B., Payne, E. C., and Chartrand, J. M. (1990). Goal instability and later life. *Psychology and Aging, 5,* 447-450.

Sanderson, C. A., and Cantor, N. (1999). A life task perspective on personality coherence: Stability versus change in tasks, goals, strategies, and outcomes. In D. Cervone and Y. Shoda (Eds.), *The coherence of personality: Social-cognitive bases of consistency, variability, and organization* (pp. 372–392). New York: Guilford.

Smith, L. C., and Robbins, S. B. (1988). Validity of the Goal Instability Scale (modified) as a predictor of adjustment in retirement-age adults. *Journal of Counseling Psychology, 35,* 325-329.

Staats, S., and Pierfelice, L. (2003). Travel: A long-range goal of retired women. *The Journal of Psychology, 137,* 483-494.

Stawski, R. S., Hershey, D. A., and Jacobs-Lawson, J. M. (2007). Goal clarity and financial planning activities as determinants of retirement savings contributions. *International Journal of Aging and Human Development, 64,* 13-32.

Thurnher, M. (1974). Goals, values, and life evaluations at the preretirement stage. *Journal of Gerontology, 29,* 85-96.

van Solinge, H. (2006). *Changing tracks: Studies on life after early retirement in the Netherlands.* The Hague: Koopman and Kraaijenbrink Publishing.

Weiner, B., and Graham, S. (1999). Attribution in personality psychology. In L. A. Pervin and O. P. John(Eds.) *The handbook of personality: Theory and research, 2nd Ed.* (pp. 605-652). New York: Guilford Press.

Wicker, F. W., Lambert, F. B., Richardson, F. C., and Kahler, J. (1984). Categorical goal hierarchies and classification of human motives. *Journal of Personality, 52,* 285-305.

Winell, M. (1987). Personal goals: The key to self-direction in adulthood. In M. E. Ford and D. H. Ford (Eds.), *Humans as self-constructing living systems: Putting the framework to work,* pp. 261-287. Hillsdale, NJ: Erlbaum Associates.

Index

A

B

C

D

E

F

G

H

I

J

K

L

Q

R

S

T

U

V

W

Y